# Springer Series on Ethics, Law, and Aging

## Series Editor
**Marshall B. Kapp, JD, MPH**
Director, Wright State University Office
of Geriatric Medicine and Gerontology
Wright State University, Dayton, OH

**Ellen Olson, MD**, is the Codirector of the Kathy and Alan C. Greenberg Center on Ethics and Geriatrics and Long-Term Care and the Director of Medical Student Education at the Jewish Home and Hospital for Aged of New York, and Assistant Professor at the Mount Sinai School of Medicine. Her publications have focused on ethics and long-term care.

**Eileen R. Chichin, DSW, RN**, is the Coordinator of the Kathy and Alan C. Greenberg Center on Ethics in Geriatrics and Long-Term Care at the Jewish Home and Hospital for Aged of New York. Her previous publications have focused on ethical issues and long-term care and on paraprofessional workers who care for the frail elderly.

**Leslie S. Libow, MD**, is the Greenwall Professor of Geriatrics and Adult Development at the Mount Sinai School of Medicine, and the Chief of Medical Services and the Codirector of the Kathy and Alan C. Greenberg Center on Ethics and Geriatrics and Long-Term Care at the Jewish Home and Hospital for Aged of New York. Dr. Libow is the editor of two books and the author of many articles on geriatric medicine. He established this nation's first training program to produce specialists in geriatric medicine and to educate generalists in the skills needed to work with the elderly, and created the concept and model of the academic nursing home.

# Controversies
## in Ethics
### in
## Long-Term Care

Ellen Olson, MD
Eileen R. Chichin, DSW, RN
Leslie S. Libow, MD

Editors

**Springer Publishing Company**

Springer Publishing Company, Inc.
536 Broadway
New York, NY 10012

Cover design by Tom Yabut
Production Editor: Joyce Noulas

00 01 02 / 5 4 3

**Library of Congress Cataloging-in-Publication Data**

Controversies in ethics in long-term-care / Ellen Olson,
    Eileen R. Chichin, Leslie S. Libow, editors.
        p.      cm.—(Springer series on Ethics, Law, and
        Aging)
    Includes bibliographical references and index.
    ISBN 0-8261-8600-9
    1. Right to die. 2. Aged—Long-term care—Moral
and ethical aspects. 3. Terminal care—Moral and
ethical aspects. 4. Senile dementia—Treatment—
Moral and ethical aspects. 5. Terminal care—Moral
and ethical aspects—Case studies. I. Olson, Ellen
(Ellen Marie), 1951- . II. Chichin, Eileen
R. III. Libow, Leslie S., 1933-
R726.C673    1994
179'.7—dc20
                                            94-23161
                                               CIP

Printed in the United States of America

# Contents

# Contributors

**Ambassador Morris B. Abram** is a lawyer, educator, civil rights activist, community leader, and diplomat. He has served in a variety of senior domestic and foreign policy positions under five American presidents of both parties. At the present time, Ambassador Abram is Chairman of the United Nations Watch in Geneva, Switzerland, which promotes the balanced, fair, and honest application of the charter principles of the United Nations within the Secretariat and the UN's other bodies, agencies, and commissions.

**David W. Bentley, MD**, is Professor of Medicine, Director of Training, and Head, Division of Geriatric Medicine at the St. Louis University Health Science Center. In addition, he is the Director of the Nursing Home Care Unit at the St. Louis Veterans Adminstration Medical Center. Dr. Bentley is the author of numerous articles on infections in the elderly.

**Philip Boyle, PhD**, is the Associate for Medical Ethics at The Hastings Center, a not-for-profit research group focusing on ethical issues in the life sciences, located in Briarcliff Manor, New York. In addition to his book, *Bioethics: The Source of Catholic Teaching*, Dr. Boyle is the author of numerous articles on ethical issues.

**Daniel Callahan, PhD**, is the cofounder and Director of The Hastings Center. He is the author of numerous articles on ethical issues, and the author or editor of 30 books, among them the critically acclaimed *Setting Limits: Medical Goals in an Aging Society*.

**Bart J. Collopy, PhD**, is Associate for Ethical Studies at the Third Age Gerontology Center and Associate Professor in the Humanities Division at Fordham University at Lincoln Center in New York City. He is also an Adjunct Associate at The Hastings Center where he served on the staff from 1987 to 1989. His recent research and writing has focused on ethical questions in institutional and community-based long-term care.

**Marianne C. Fahs, PhD, MPH**, is Associate Professor and Director, Division of Health Economics at the Mount Sinai School of Medicine in New York City. She is the author of numerous articles on cost effectiveness analysis and prevention services, and has served on several national advisory committees.

**Harvey Finkelstein, MS**, is the President and Chief Executive Officer of the Jewish Home and Hospital for Aged of New York. His previous publications and presentations have focused on both long-term care and public health issues.

**Jack P. Freer, MD, FACP**, is Clinical Assistant Professor of Medicine (Division of General Internal Medicine and Division of Geriatrics-Gerontology), University of Buffalo. Dr. Freer teaches medical ethics at the School of Medicine and Biomedical Sciences, and is Medical Director of the Millard Fillmore Hospital Skilled Nursing Facility. He has published widely on issues of medical ethics.

**Ann C. Hurley, RN, DNSc**, is the Associate Director for Education and Program Evaluation at the Geriatric Research, Education, and Clinical Center the Edith Nourse Rogers Memorial Veterans Hospital in Bedford, Massachusetts. She is the author of several articles on ethical issues, diabetes, and Alzheimer's disease.

**Bruce Jennings, MA**, is a political scientist by training. He is the Executive Director of The Hastings Center in Briarcliff Manor, New York. He has written or edited nine books and numerous articles on ethical issues in medicine and public policy.

**John J. LaPuma, MD**, is a consultant in Clinical Ethics at Lutheran General Hospital and Clinical Associate Professor of Medicine at the University of Chicago. A practicing physician, Dr LaPuma is the author of numerous articles on ethical issues in medicine, and co-author with David Schiedermayer of *Ethics Consultation: A Practical Guide*.

**Margaret A. Mahoney, RN, PhD**, is a consultant to the Geriatric Research, Education, and Clinical Center the Edith Nourse Rogers Memorial Veterans Hospital in Bedford, Massachusetts, and Visiting Professor at Northeastern University in Boston. She has worked and published in the area of family decision-making for advanced Alzheimer's patients, and the nurse's role in surrogate decision-making.

**Ladislaw Volicer, MD, PhD**, is the Clinical Director of the Geriatric Research, Education, and Clinical Center the Edith Nourse Rogers Memorial Veterans Hospital in Bedford, Massachusetts, and Professor of Pharmacology and Psychiatry and Assistant Professor of Medicine at Boston University. Dr. Volicer has developed innovative models of providing care in end-stage Alzheimer's disease and has published numerous articles on clinical issues and terminal care of late-stage and terminal care for individuals with dementia.

# Acknowledgments

This volume and the conference on which it is based are undertakings of the Kathy and Alan C. Greenberg Center on Ethics in Geriatrics and Long-Term Care at the Jewish Home and Hospital for Aged of New York (JHHA) and are the collaborative effort of a number of people. Although they cannot all be mentioned by name, there are some who deserve special note.

A major debt of gratitude is owed to the Frederick and Amelia Schimper Foundation, and in particular, Mr. Myles A. Cane for their generous financial assistance for both the conference and this book. We are most grateful to the Board of Trustees and administration of JHHA who have consistently supported the work of the Center on Ethics. The Hastings Center offered valuable advice during the planning and development of the conference, and we were honored to have them as the conference cosponsor.

Special thanks must go to the New York Academy of Medicine, particularly Martha Klapp, for the prominent role it played in the conference. JHHA staff members, especially Estelle Cooper, Frances Feltz, Liz Friedman, and Harriet Kriegel, provided invaluable assistance, as did our colleagues at the Mount Sinai Medical Center, particularly Linda Weiss.

We are grateful to Rosalie Kane for her role in our conference. Her presence markedly enhanced its quality.

JHHA's Center on Ethics has been fortunate in attracting students who have worked most effectively with us in internship positions. Two of these students, Brita Kube of the University of Michigan and Elizabeth Zito of Columbia University, were instrumental in the success of the conference and the development of this volume, while Joan Bromfield of the Columbia School of Social Work assisted with the preparation of the manuscript. We are also grateful to Helene Meyers, the administrator of our Manhattan facility, for her helpful comments on the final drafts of our manuscript.

We would like to recognize the early contributions of Drs. Christine Cassel and Richard Neufeld in helping to establish the ethics programs at JHHA.

And finally, we must acknowledge the members of various health-related disciplines at JHHA and the residents for whom they care. Our work with them provided inspiration for both the conference and this book. Perhaps more important, they continue to inspire us daily as we work together to face the challenges presented by these current controversies in ethics and long-term care.

# Foreword

There is an ancient Chinese curse that says, "May you live in interesting times." Today the health care system in America is very interesting indeed, and in many respects it does seem to be cursed. We see the strengths of our system in our first-rate facilities and our superbly trained and dedicated health professionals. We see the growing power of medical science and technology in the struggle against premature death, curable disease, and preventable disability. And yet we wonder if we have the capacity to manage health care delivery and expenditure in a rational, efficient way without eroding or sacrificing the high quality of care most Americans have come to expect.

Moreover, we see the injustice and discrimination of our current health insurance system, and we see the moral imperative of extending universal coverage and access. Beyond that, many look forward to an even more fundamental reorientation of health care delivery, emphasizing primary and preventive services, to move from what is today mainly a *sickness care* system into a true *health care* system. And yet again, we wonder if it is possible to muster the political will and leadership to move away from the comforting familiarity of the status quo, warts and all, into a land of new organizational structures and untested reforms.

As this is being written, in early 1994, hopes and expectations are running high about the possibilities of systematic health reform in the United States. More ink has been spilled on this topic in the past 12 months than in the preceding 10 years.

But despite all of the commentary and high-profile attention, current public dialogue about the future of health care is notable for what it omits. It has virtually shunted aside the entire problem of chronic and long-term care. It has ignored the serious ethical quandaries associated with health care rationing; when rationing is discussed at all, it is turned into a political football.

Finally, the health reform debate has yet to lock horns in any direct way with an unresolved moral debate that has been simmering and churning in our society for many years. I refer to the issues of the sanctity of and quality of life. When, if ever, is life no longer worth living for the individual? When, if ever, should society refuse to bear the expense of prolonging or sustaining life through artificial means? These questions cannot be dismissed easily or simply by remarking that it is impossible—or morally inappropriate—to put a price tag on human life. These questions are profound—and profoundly difficult ones—they go to the heart of what we understand by the meaning of human life and the human good; they point out the enduring tension between the moral claims of the individual and those of the community.

Long-term care, rationing, and quality of life are now coming to the forefront of the study of bioethics, and that is a most welcome and overdue development. Deep and careful moral reflection requires patience and is the work of many hands. These questions will not be resolved this year or next year or the year after that. We have before us the slow, laborious task of listening to one another, learning from one another, and plumbing the depths of our minds and hearts.

This volume, growing out of a stimulating conference convened in 1993 under the auspices of the Kathy and Alan C. Greenberg Center on Ethics in Geriatrics and Long-Term Care at the Jewish Home and Hospital for Aged, provides a welcome and timely impetus to get on with that task. The chapters here represent some of the best-informed and most rigorous thinking we have on the ethical dimensions of long-term care, from the varying perspectives of patients and families, state-of-the-art medical care in such areas as pain management and antibiotic therapy, hands-on caregivers in the nursing home setting, and public policy.

This book has the courage to break silence on the need for more attention to long-term care in bioethics and public policy, on the problem of rationing, and on the ubiquitous nature of value judgments regarding the sanctity of and quality of life. It has the considerable merit of not only opening up the conversation on these neglected topics but also showing their interconnection with one another. We won't settle on a rational and just long-term care policy in this country until we learn to face up to the problem of just health care rationing. And we won't, I expect, get our priorities straight until we reexamine precisely what we, as individuals and as a society, ought to expect from medicine and health care employed in service of human flourishing and the human good.

Everyone reading this volume will come away better informed and enlightened on these questions. And no one reading it will be able, in good conscience, to avoid these questions any longer.

BRUCE JENNINGS, MA

# Introduction and Overview

Nowhere in the U.S. health care system are ethical issues as pervasive as they are in long-term care and care of the frail elderly, wherever they reside. With shrinking resources on the one hand and demands for technologically advanced life-extending treatments on the other, health care professionals—and indeed the entire nation—face increasingly critical ethical issues regarding care of the elderly. In this book a number of ethicists and long-term care professionals discuss many of the particular problems associated with ethical decision making. This volume should provide valuable assistance to those who work in the long-term care setting and hope to respond to these issues more effectively and more humanely.

The field of biomedical ethics has come alive largely because of the changing population. This "new demography" pushes us toward a new kind of medicine. At the center of the issue is the balance among morality, medicine, and money. Each day, those involved in providing long-term care struggle with numerous dilemmas, such as determining how a patient's wishes can be carried out in the absence of advance directives. How can the autonomy and privacy of frail elderly be preserved when they are so dependent upon others for their most basic needs? Do most elderly really desire advance directives and seek autonomy? Much evidence reveals advance directives to be a creation of the young on behalf of an unwilling elderly population. Under what circumstances can or should treatment be withheld or withdrawn? How do we minimize the anguish of patients, family members, and staff when such measures are taken?

Health care providers in long-term care regularly face a struggle between their roles as clinicians and the roles they are being asked to fill as economists for society at large. For example, as a member of a community or institutional committee, a physician, nurse, or social worker may find it logical and necessary to cut costs, to limit staff from whatever discipline. However, as clinicians, their responsibility as advocates for patients is paramount. At times, of course, this may mean assisting a patient to achieve a goal contrary to most of their prior training; that is, to cease treatment in the traditional sense of medicine and technology and to begin to assist the patient, the family, and the staff in the final days of life. It takes a highly skilled and knowledgeable clinician to reach a conclusion that classical medicine can do no more.

As noted in a recent editorial in the *New England Journal of Medicine* (Kassirer, 1993), health care has not been so much at center stage for many years, perhaps for many decades, perhaps not even since the beginning of the 20th century. Major changes, therefore, will definitely occur, some good and some more negative for the elderly.

New initiatives will emerge from Washington and will most likely have little to do with long-term care. In fact, it is anticipated that there will be some sharp limits on government funding for long-term care. Public expenditures will be capped, and those with private funds will be able to buy more services. There will be a decreased use of hospitals as nursing homes become, in part, the site of what was previously the hospital domain. In addition, there will probably be a cap on all types of dollars spent by the government, through Medicare or Medicaid, for the elderly. But basic health needs will be supplied to all and new things will be given to make people feel a little better. Medications will probably be paid for, and psychiatric care may be better reimbursed.

What do all of the people want with regard to their health care? Too little is known to us and to government. However well intentioned, too many actions by government, state, and federal agencies occur without the basic facts being available. Often, these actions are directed at saving money.

For example, we have placed some hope in the concept of advance directives. We are encouraged to ask people of all ages, but especially the elderly, to write about their treatment preferences in case of incapacity at some future time. It *sounds* like a good idea.

There is an enthusiasm about the importance of choosing proxies and surrogates so that others will know what you want should you become decisionally impaired. But interventions at the end of life are generally limited by advance directives. Thus, by encouraging their use, we may, in some way be serving as economists. After all, if everyone has a living will and a proxy, it is likely that the cost of health care to society will be less. That's probably good, but we must be extremely cautious about this, especially with respect to more vulnerable, poorer populations, who may be encouraged to limit their treatment as a cost-containment measure while those with great wealth are able to buy more extensive treatment.

What have older people said about advance directives? Perhaps 10% of American elderly have advance directives. In most nursing homes, less than 10% of the residents have advance directives. The fact is, very few people in general, and elderly in particular, have chosen to execute advance directives.

Are they dangerous, these advance directives? I consider them important, although potentially dangerous. A case in point is an 83-year-old, fully competent translator and lawyer. She wrote an advance directive stipulating that she wanted no tubes, no respirators, or the like. One year later, she agreed to colon surgery for a suspected cancer. The night before surgery I saw her at the hospital. She said, "It's all in God's hands."

Fortunately, it turned out to be an abscess, and we were all quite happy. About a day or two later, however, she suffered a respiratory arrest. Should she have been intubated at that time in an attempt to save her life? Some will say, "Of course," and others will say, "Well, how could you?" In fact, a great uproar occurred around this situation. The surgeon, who, by chance, was on hand when the arrest occurred, called the team, and she was subsequently intubated. For a period of time, she was on a respirator. During that time there was much consternation at both the hospital and the long-term care facility she considered her home.

The story has an interesting ending. The tubes were removed; the patient survived. She was fine. Three weeks later, when I asked, "What do you think about what happened?" She said, "I guess, in my advance directive [she called it 'my living will'] I didn't say I shouldn't be intubated in this exact situation, but in any case, Doctor, I was ready to die." Clearly, we must be aware of the pitfalls of advance directives while we applaud them.

Another issue of concern with respect to frail older people is that of informed consent. We tell older persons all about the risks of and gains to be accrued from procedures such as surgery, medications, transfer to the hospital, transfer to the nursing home, and rehabilitation. Then, most often, they consent to these procedures. They sign something. But is this ill, frail older person really absorbing the full impact? Is this really an informed consent? Has the clinician possibly prejudiced the presentation, knowingly or unknowingly, through the manner in which he or she described the procedure? I believe that, for the frail elderly, informed consent is a shaky concept. The concept that I like to call informed trust is worth considering: we inform, but the patient's signature takes on less meaning. The clinician still assumes responsibility, especially in a moral sense, for the action to be taken. In other words, trust is placed in the clinician and in what is being done.

Yet another issue unique to the long-term care setting—both nursing homes and home care programs—involves the clinical staff. The involvement of these individuals with those for whom they care is very different in long-term care from that in the hospital. The hospital is a 7–10-day stay, and the patient is gone, hopefully discharged to home. The nursing home and home care represent a thousand-day stay. Obviously, the staff members in these latter programs—the nursing assistant in particular—become surrogate families to their residents and clients and, accordingly, become deeply involved emotionally. Therefore, any decision that involves an action as profound as the termination of life-sustaining treatment must involve the surrogate family. One hopes that it usually does. This issue and several others particularly problematic in the long-term care setting will be addressed in this book.

## FORMAT OF THE BOOK

The chapters in this volume are based on presentations given at a conference sponsored by the Schimper Foundation and organized by the Greenberg Center on Ethics of the Jewish Home and Hospital for Aged of New York. Each chapter focuses on an issue particularly relevant to long-term care. Following each chapter is a case derived from our clinical experience that reflects some of the issues addressed in the chapter. Each case has suggested answers and approaches that readers may want to consider as they begin to address the issues that are presented. All of the cases involve ethical issues, and many also focus on hands-on, clinical aspects of care. Accordingly, this book will be useful to practitioners in the long-term care field who regularly grapple with these challenges and also to students in a variety of health-related disciplines who are contemplating careers in long-term care.

Chapter 1 focuses on the role of advance directives as they relate to older people. Some feel that all of the treatment decision-making problems related to decisionally impaired older persons will be solved in the future if people execute some form of advance directive prior to experiencing cognitive decline. However, advance directives may be a poor substitute for better patient–physician communication and increased dialogue within families. And what of the frail elderly without advance directives and without family? How are decisions to be made for them? Dr. John LaPuma, in his chapter "Are Advance Directives the Answer for the Frail Elderly?" draws on his clinical experience and the minimal empirical evidence available to describe the current status of advance directives as they pertain to our present population of frail elderly. In addition, he suggests how long-term care staff can best deal with issues related to advance directives in their practice.

In the second chapter, Dr. Philip Boyle discusses one of the major challenges of long-term care: issues associated with cultural diversity among staff and residents in nursing homes. The excitement of America is contained in its variety of cultures, but so is a special challenge. Is cultural diversity an impediment to a caring environment? Are there other factors—racial, socioeconomic, and differences in levels of education—that contribute to conflicts between long-term care staff and the people entrusted to their care? Dissimilarities between caregivers and patients may lead to serious implications for both groups, resulting in situations as benign as simple misunderstandings or as serious as verbal or physical abuse. Dr. Boyle describes the impact of cultural diversity, particularly religious differences, on the residents and staff of nursing homes and the implications of these differences on day-to-day interactions.

Chapter 3 focuses on the effect that treatment termination has on the caregiving staff. The termination of life-prolonging treatment clearly has profound implications for any individual who has chosen to forgo such a treatment. However, others markedly affected by a home care client's or nursing home resident's treatment termination are the health care providers. In long-term care settings, the intensity and longevity of relationships between patients and health care providers result in caregivers becoming, in effect, surrogate families to those for whom they care. How do these staff members perceive their roles when treatment is terminated? What is the impact on them of caring for someone who is dying as a result of treatment termination? How can we best support the resident's "natural" or traditional family and those members of the nursing home "family" or those paid caregivers in the home who become surrogate family? Where should our efforts be directed, and how can a facility's or program's resources best be utilized to help all concerned deal with this difficult issue?

Dr. Eileen Chichin discusses in Chapter 3 the impact on family and staff when a nursing home resident opts to have life-sustaining treatment withheld or withdrawn. Findings obtained from a pilot study of a nursing home staff involved in caring for residents who have died as a result of treatment termination is discussed, in addition to interventions to support both family members and health care providers through this difficult process.

All members of the health care team are affected by a resident's decision to terminate treatment, but physicians have their own unique set of experiences. Many physicians are still grappling with their own loss of autonomy in end-of-life treatment decision making. In addition, some are distressed by the idea of not providing classical medical treatment to patients who are chronically but not terminally ill.

In Chapter 4, Dr. Ellen Olson discusses the impact of treatment termination on physicians in the long-term care setting, and suggests interventions to help the physician cope with this changing role and also to understand the idiosyncratic nature of what constitutes a good death.

Dr. Olson also focuses on others markedly affected by treatment termination decisions—the family members of those who opt to have treatment withheld or withdrawn. Even in those situations in which family members recognize that treatment termination is the resident's wish, they are often markedly troubled by the impending death of another family member. One question that often arises is who really is the "patient" in these situations—the nursing home resident whose treatment is being withheld or withdrawn, or the family member who is severely affected by this process? In discussing the impact of treatment termination on families, Dr. Olson suggests interventions to assist these families.

Another issue that assumes prominence in the long-term care arena will be addressed by Dr. Bart Collopy in Chapter 5, "Home versus Nursing Home: Getting Beyond the Differences." The increasing dependency that is the usual concomitant of old age often causes frail elderly and their families to seek community-based or institutional long-term care services. A number of factors influence both access to these services and the experience of individuals who utilize them. These factors range from the individual level to the societal level and include the ability to pay for services in one setting (as opposed to the other) and the loss of some personal rights and autonomy that may occur with institutionalization. For individuals without sufficient financial resources, care at home may be limited, but remaining at home may be the only place to avoid the regulatory influences over end-of-life treatment decisions, especially in the frail individual without capacity. At times and with available funding, home care can be arranged to be equal or superior to institutional care. Available are rehabilitative therapists, nurses, pharmacists, physicians, clergy, and one's own surroundings and family. Can "family" autonomy and rights be preserved without deleterious effects on an institution, its staff, and society in general? Where should people live out their last days—in their own homes, where they may be less safe but retain a higher degree of autonomy, or in a nursing home, where they will be protected but will relinquish some personal freedom? Are a person's rights more protected at home or in the nursing home? In discussing these issues, Dr. Collopy places them in the larger framework of the meaning of frailty and advanced old age.

In Chapter 6, Dr. Ann Hurley discusses comfort care: "What to Do after Deciding to Do No More." The provision of comfort care to those who are dying is perhaps the most significant role a caregiver can play in another's dying process. Providing such care may be equally important for both health care providers and those for whom they care when the dying process occurs as a result of

treatment termination. Withholding or withdrawing life-prolonging treatment is considered repugnant by many health care professionals, who perceive such acts to be antithetical to their mission. Nonetheless, acceptable medical practice, current law, and
respect for autonomy dictate that, when an individual so chooses,
such treatments can be stopped. In those situations, health care
providers who previously have taken an active role in the preservation of life may feel that they are now deliberately causing death.
Educating these individuals regarding the importance of their
roles in both the provision of comfort care and respect for patient autonomy may, to some degree, ameliorate the distress they
experience. A better understanding of what constitutes comfort
care may also be helpful in this process because staff often insist
that treatment measures be continued in the name of comfort
care when these particular treatment measures may also prolong
the dying process.

In this chapter, Dr. Hurley describes the continuing role for
health care professionals when life-prolonging treatment is terminated in end-stage dementia, focusing on the replacement of high-
tech care with high-touch care. The latter involves nurses, physicians, social workers, and the entire team.

Another issue related to comfort care is the use of antibiotics.
Traditionally, antibiotics have been administered to patients with
advanced dementias who develop intercurrent infections because
this treatment is seen as noninvasive and simple to administer.
The question arises as to whether antibiotics should be employed
at all in these situations; is it better simply to "let nature take its
course" ?

In some life-threatening conditions, the use of antibiotics can
have a twofold effect. That is, although antibiotics are a treatment, the treatment relieves symptoms and, in so doing, provides
comfort. When does the use of antibiotics constitute treatment,
and when is it comfort care? Should poor prognoses influence
decisions to withhold antibiotics? In their chapter, Dr. Jack Freer
and Dr. David Bentley discuss the unique role that antibiotics
may play when persons with end-stage dementia develop infec-
tious processes that, in any other situation, would automatically
be treated with antibiotics. Drs. Freer and Bentley also outline
parameters that may be used in making a decision to use this
form of treatment.

Chapters 8 and 9 focus on an area of particular concern not only to those who live and work in the long-term care setting but also to policymakers: the ethical and economic issues associated with providing care at the end of life to those suffering from dementing illnesses.

In Chapter 8, Dr. Daniel Callahan discusses the ethical issues and possible imperatives to continue treatment associated with providing life-sustaining treatment to persons with end-stage dementia. Is it ethical to develop a policy stating when care can be terminated? When terminal dementia renders a person incontinent, unable to recognize loved ones, unable to speak and unable to swallow, should medical interventions continue when they only serve to reverse the intercurrent illness but not the disease itself?

Given the projected increases in our elderly population, can we as a society afford to continue to provide unlimited medical care for growing numbers of severely demented elderly? What are the implications of this for other disabled and vulnerable populations if the elderly claim an increasing proportion of our health care expenditures? In Chapter 9, Dr. Marianne Fahs, a health economist, discusses the economic issues associated with providing life-sustaining treatment to persons with end-stage dementia.

Clearly, all of the above-described issues are paramount to those who care for the frail elderly in nursing homes and home care programs. To date, few, if any, books have addressed these concerns, nor suggested interventions to begin to address them. We hope that this book's readers find it useful as they strive to enhance the lives and ease the deaths of those for whom they care.

LESLIE S. LIBOW, M.D.

## REFERENCES

Kassirer, T. H. (1993). Medicine at center stage. *New England Journal of Medicine, 328*(17), 1268–1269.

# 1

# Are Advance Directives the Answer for the Frail Elderly?

*John La Puma*

The short answer to the question of whether advance directives are the solution to concerns about medical decision making for the frail elderly is that they are better than some things but not many.

Written advance directives as they are presently utilized and understood do not serve us well. A significant body of evidence suggests that the elderly in general and the nursing home population in particular stand together with the vast majority of Americans in their reluctance to complete written advance directives (Diamond, Jernigan, Mosley, Messina, & McKeown, 1989). The frail elderly who have designated someone else, usually a family member, to make decisions for them are unlikely to know that the correlation between what they want and what their agent would choose is not much better than chance (Schneiderman, Pearlman, Kaplan, Anderson, & Rosenberg, 1992).

Some people believe that advance directives are actually dangerous for the frail elderly, who may be especially unable to voice questions or concerns about their use and interpretation once illness strikes. To the extent that advance directives will be used to limit needed or desired care, to substitute for doctor–patient dialogue, and to replace discussions of "shoulds" with discussions of requirements, advance directives are indeed dangerous for the elderly.

There is a possibility, however, that the debate about advance directives and proxy decision making is being framed in the wrong way. The real debate is not about rights, and the right to die, but instead, about the quality of life and relationships in a medical and social community. Principles of medical professionalism, combined and balanced with the principle of patient autonomy, can help answer the questions about quality of life that advance directives raise.

## ADVANCE DIRECTIVES: PITFALLS

Experience to date with advance directives suggests that writing things down does not seem always to help. General instructions about how patients want to be treated do not seem to be related to their specific feelings about specific future treatments (Schneiderman et al., 1992). Experience in ethics consultation (La Puma & Scheidermayer, 1994) suggests that different patients mean different things when they fill out written advance directives and that physicians often do not know what to do when confronted with them. The most important, determinative factor of whether a patient's advance directive is respected seems to be whether the patient's physician agrees with the patient's decision (personal communication, J. Lynn to JL, April 29, 1993).

Particular patient cases illustrate the problems with relying on advance directives for health care planning for patients. A case in point involves a patient who was thought to be demented:

> An 81-year-old widower had cardiomyopathy and renal failure. His girlfriend lived nearby and visited nightly. He worked as a professional bookmaker and traveled annually to Las Vegas. He had not seen his two sisters in 8 years. His girlfriend insisted on no dialysis; his sisters insisted that he should be dialyzed. The social worker reported the girlfriend's complaint that dialysis would "cost too much." The cardiologist asked the ethics consultant, "Given the family dispute and girlfriend's apparent financial conflict, what is the proper course of action regarding dialysis?"
>
> On examination, the patient appeared mildly confused. He said, however, "I'm not crazy—Don't let them tell you that! I want to live as long as I can." Dialysis disturbed and frightened him, but he said he might not mind as long as he could still go to Las Vegas. The consultant convened a late-night family meeting. The girlfriend complained that the sisters were uninvolved and opportunistic. She called them "vultures" and ac-

cused them of being interested only in the patient's estate. The sisters denied this, saying that she was "the vulture." Near the meeting's end, the girlfriend pulled a legal document from her purse and asked, "Can this help?"

The consultant took the proxy form naming the girlfriend as the patient's health-care agent to his bedside. It had been completed during the hospitalization, and the most restrictive treatment plan had been checked. The patient was surprised. "She did that. I signed it, but she did that. Let me talk about it with her." He had recently revised his will, giving his girlfriend much of his $400,000 estate.

The ethics consultant recommended accepting the patient's own present-day choice to proceed with dialysis and discussing the advance directive again when the patient regained full decision-making capacity. After dialysis, the patient improved and returned home.[1]

This case shows that appropriate medical treatment can sometimes be overlooked in our legalistic attention to written advance directives. Advance directives here were a flag for discussion of proxy decision making and patient autonomy, as well as an impetus to review optional treatment. At their best, advance directives can be flags in the care of the frail elderly, and offer a general notion about care and treatment near the end of life.

## WILL EDUCATION ABOUT ADVANCE DIRECTIVES HELP THE DECISIONALLY CAPABLE FRAIL ELDERLY?

Educational attempts among physicians and patients to increase the numbers of advance directives are nearly always noble, but given the controversy about directives' helpfulness, the goals of educational attempts should be clearly defined before they are attempted. Any education should be about communication, not simply documentation. Education about care near the end of life is likely to be successful only within the context of an established, continuing doctor–patient relationship.

Help for the frail elderly and for many other patients lies in a stronger, more communicative, more personal understanding between doctor and patient. It also lies in the merging of the principles of medical professionalism with the principle of patient autonomy. Professionalism must be balanced with autonomy, and doctors, nurses, and social workers must take the lead in learning about our patients' values and strengthening our relationships with patients. This mandate will become even more important, given the coming challenges to patient well-being that managed care and the Health Security Act of 1993 will create and pose (Nash, 1994).

## DO PROXIES REPRESENT PATIENT AUTONOMY?

Too often, when a patient has executed a health-care proxy, the patient's autonomy is expressed in a document as the health-care agent's choice, not the patient's choice, whether patient designated or legally designated, and it is this form of patient autonomy that frustrates providers most. For example: An 80-year-old hypertensive woman has multiinfarct dementia but can understand and respond appropriately to simple commands and recognize her grandchildren and nursing home attendants. She enters the hospital for the second time in 5 months with an elevated temperature and lethargy. Her daughter asked the admitting physician who cared for the patient during the previous recent admission to "let her go," saying that the patient would not want "to live like this." She told the nurse that the nursing home would no longer accept Medicaid and that she could not afford to pay her mother's bills.

There is little indication of how this 80-year-old patient would want the doctor to act. As previously noted (Schneiderman et al., 1992), proxy conjecture of how a patient would act or of how the patient would want the health-care agent to act is not significantly related to how the patient would actually act. The doctor cannot hope to respect the patient's autonomy by talking with the agent in this case.

Both the doctor and the agent are now caught in an administrative bind in which personal, medical, financial, and ethical problems are all wrapped up together. The agent's frustrated attempt to escape her own burden while trying to represent the patient's wishes is clear. Can the agent keep straight the difference between treatments that are technically indicated and those that are financially available? Can the agent synthesize the patient's values, escape her own emotional and financial burdens, and avoid a "conflict of interest" with her mother? Can patient autonomy really be represented by what the agent wants? Could advance directives as we currently understand them—duly recorded but often undiscussed treatment choices, goals, and objectives—offer insight about how to care for this patient?

Cases like that of this unfortunate woman do not suggest a return to paternalism, something that no humane physician should wish. Nor do they negate the importance of patient and family values. Indeed, they heighten this importance, as these values are not understood in this case. Cases like this do make us wonder why we value patient autonomy, as expressed through advance directives, the way we do.

## CAN ETHICS CONSULTATION HELP IN DIFFICULT CASES?

However useful ethics consultants and ethics committees can be in bringing to the forefront important information and issues involving particular cases, they cannot reverse the inherent weaknesses of advance directives or surrogate decision making. In addition, formalized ethics consultations tend to be very time-consuming and are not always covered by Medicare or Medicaid, the major sources of reimbursement for most nursing home services. The absence of an appropriate financial recognition of the importance of patients' value systems is part of the reason that most long-term care facilities and hospitals still do not have an ethics consultant on staff.

## DO THE FRAIL ELDERLY VALUE AUTONOMY?

An expanded vision of respect for autonomy with the elderly calls for balancing an understanding of patient preference, to the extent it is offered or can be elicited, with an understanding of proxy preference, and with the physician's integrated assessment of the medical circumstances as a whole. It has been suggested that the definition of autonomy needs to be modified to address the preference of an older population for shared decision making rather than individual autonomy (Kapp, 1991). Many elderly patients seem to desire less personal involvement in medical decision making, giving their families and physicians a larger role in making these decisions than do younger patients (Biesecker, 1988; High, 1988; Wagner, 1984; Wetle, Levkoff, Cwikel, & Rosen, 1988).

Even if the frail elderly did highly or absolutely value autonomy, purely autonomous decision making is probably impossible to achieve. Some philosophers believe that communitarian[2] concerns vitiate an elderly patient's authority to decide for herself (Blustein, 1993). Indeed, purely autonomous decision making is probably undesirable for an interdependent, growing community. Loewy (1992) writes: "Autonomy does not exist in a vacuum but is developed, enunciated, and ultimately exercised in the embrace of others. To deny the social nexus of autonomy is threatening both to the social nexus and to autonomy" (p. 1976). As individual as autonomy is, it exists within the network of community.

Lastly, the elderly and their physicians may not be consistent enough in their thinking to make the same health care choices, even in the same circumstances, from one day to the next. For example, Malloy, Wigton, Meeske, & Tape (1992) found that among 201 persons (mean age, 76 years) in Omaha, 155 (77%) changed their minds about whether to accept or reject CPR, mechanical ventilation, and tube feeding, based simply on the way the treatment was described. Two-thirds of these 155 changed their minds four times or more.

## NO ADVANCE DIRECTIVES AND NO PROXY: HOW SHOULD MEDICAL DECISIONS BE MADE?

The frail elderly, the medically indigent, the demented, and the institutionalized are among our most vulnerable citizens and patients. Who will make sure advantage is not taken of them? Who will watch out for their health and assets?

The short answer to this question is, It will have to be done case by case. The longer answer lies in two very different realms: how health care is financed and doctors are paid and why diverse multi-cultural views of community in the United States are so important. Each can be described briefly.

Medical practice appears to be influenced by financial incentives. Positive incentives to prescribe or administer additional treatment have, in part, been responsible for the enormous increase in Medicare spending over its nearly two decades. Positive incentives to withhold or withdraw care have been equally effective in reducing health care expenditures within vertically integrated managed-care organizations. If physicians were better compensated for discussions with patients regarding their values and preferences for health care, then patients' expected survival might be more equitably balanced with quality-of-life considerations and patient preference by those who are charged with caring for the patient.

Communities and cultures within the United States are more diverse and heterogeneous than the male, middle-class Caucasian community that dominates medicine. Still, how each of us views our society's most vulnerable members varies from town to town and region to region, not just class to class. Fortunately, views of vulnerable others have a baseline and minimum standard of behavior: rules of law. The law protects and respects the personal nature of any given patient's values. When these values are undiscoverable or uncertain, reference to the way patients were raised, what they used to be like and what they used to like have intellectual and emotional appeal as these references often categorize an individual into an ethnic or cultural "type." Even these personal details, however, are usually not specific enough to the clinical circumstance at hand to be decisive. Family input into this process, despite the previously described inaccuracies of family decision making, can sometimes enhance and further personalize this third-person approach to decision making. A redefinition of family, with the frail elderly patient in mind, is needed for such decision making to be morally based. The surrogate laws of most states do not include close friends, nursing home aides, cousins, and great-nieces, who often provide care and become family, even to those residents with "closer" blood relatives. Family members are people you love and people who love you in a way that carries responsibility, accountability, and interdependence. The reasons for these feelings and duties are irrelevant; the feelings and duties themselves are relevant.

## IS AN IDEALIZED FORM OF THE DOCTOR-PATIENT RELATIONSHIP ALL THAT IS LEFT?

If it indeed is true that written advance directives, although written, are not enough; that proxy and family decision making, practical and well-intentioned as it often is, is not enough; and that ethics consultations, as helpful but as time-consuming, and highly specialized as they are, are also unavailable to most patients and

families in long-term care, then what is left? Can policies that try
to set up shared goals rely on situational judgment, and negotiated, honest, thorough discussions of care ever be implemented,
or do such policies just represent an idealized form of the doctor–patient and institution–health care worker relationship?

Every physician can still make a difference, and in long-term
care especially, the potential for relationships that are characterized more by socialization than by episodic, in- and out-of-office
visits is promising and good. Negotiated discussions of patient
values can begin with the simple asking of one question (the least-
asked question in medical ethics): Why?

The question of relational medical ethics is being asked of the
elderly because of the major demographic transition now taking
place among our aging population. To address the ethical dilemmas that advance directives attempt to answer (though in a mech-
anistic, impersonal way) and that proxy decision making tries to
address (though again impersonally and sometimes without attention to the individual patient) we need a new medical ethic.

We need a new medical ethic to answer questions of autonomy
and justice, and one that is less focused on death and dying and
more focused on quality of life and living. This medical ethic
would view patients less as atomistic, separate individuals and
more as members of families, communities, particular cultures
or religious or ethnic groups, or however patients themselves
define themselves. This new medical ethic would focus less on
hierarchies and rules and forms and more on the connection that
we can have to understand one another. In short, we need a medical ethic that is grounded in respect for clinical circumstances as
a whole, not just patient autonomy and have at its core a fundamental understanding that doctors and patients are not so
different.

Both doctors and patients are members of families and of communities. The doctor–patient relationship is grounded in a common understanding of the ultimate interrelationship of personal,
familial, and societal good. The expertise and concern with which
physicians are trained and the kindness and compassion they can
show provide reassurances that this relationship can be a reality.
Patients and families want to be cared for by such physicians in
communities that value them as much when they are old as when
they are young, regardless of whether they can speak for
themselves.

Yet the social nexus of the doctor-patient relationship, the foundation of modern medical ethics, is being tested by a quake of historic proportions. When a patient enters a new institution and is no longer cared for by the physicians with whom he or she has a relationship of caring, feelings of abandonment and loss abound, on both sides. "Who will take care of me when I leave the hospital/retirement community?" too often ends with "I'm sorry, I don't know. I don't go to that nursing home." Many such breaking and broken relationships exist today. More will occur, as patients, dependents, employers, and the government shop for the best price and adequate quality, and payers effectively decide which relationships can continue.

The way for patients to achieve their own goals for their health and for their families to achieve their goals for patients who cannot speak for themselves is not through additional federal, state, or local regulation or through medical directives, living wills, or proxy forms. It is especially not through a legally prescribed hierarchy of decision makers (Menikoff, Sachs, & Siegler, 1992; Simpson, 1993) beginning with the "next of kin," as if it were a decision about organs and tissues at funeral homes.

The way for patients to achieve their goals is by strengthening their relationships with their families and with their physicians together and by clinicians doing the hard and good work that every clinician can do. This work now includes a relational advocacy. How will decisions for this patient affect the patient's family and the patient's place in the community? Every clinician should search, not just for patients' choices but for their reasons for those choices.

Every patient wants a personal, satisfying, encouraging, reassuring relationship with his or her physician. Every doctor wants to care for patients with the good judgment he or she has tried to develop, with the knowledge of the uncertainty of disease, and with the certainty that none of us lives forever. Respect for patients, especially vulnerable patients like the demented, the disabled, and the medically indigent, implies more physician involvement in this relationship, not less (Loewy, 1992).

Patient autonomy and patient proxies must now be thought of in terms of reasons, families, and community. A balancing of patient autonomy with other ethical principles and a stronger doctor-patient understanding seek to give medical care and medical ethics a new focus on quality of life. In this era of medical cost containment, the strength of the doctor–patient relationship is in learning about patients' values and the reasons for their choices and how those choices are made within the family and community.

## NOTES

1. Adapted from La Puma, 1991.
2. Communitarian concerns are described as a view that sees dignity and self-respect "in the web of human relationships that constitutes our social identity: in short, in community" (Moody, 1992, p. 181).

## REFERENCES

Beisecker, A. E. (1988). Aging and the desire for information and input in medical decisions: Patient consumerism in medical encounters. *Gerontologist, 28*(3), 330–335.

Blustein, J. (1993). The family in medical decision-making. *Hastings Center Report, 23*(3), 6–13.

Cohen-Mansfield, J., Rabinovich, B. A., Lipson, S., Fein, A., Gerber, B., Weisman, S., Pawlson, L. G. (1991). The decision to execute a durable power of attorney for health care and preferences regarding the utilization of life-sustaining treatments in nursing home residents. *The Archives of Internal Medicine, 151*, 289–294.

Diamond, E. L., Jernigan, J. A., Mosley, R. A., Messina, V. & McKeown, R.A. (1989). Decision-making ability and advance directive preferences in nursing home patients and proxies. *Gerontologist, 29*(5), 615–621.

High, D. (1988). All in the family: Extended autonomy and expectations in surrogate health care decision-making. *Gerontologist, 28 (suppl)*, 46–51.

Kapp, M. B. (1991). Health care decision making by the elderly: I get by with a little help from my family. *Gerontologist, 5*(31), 619–623.

La Puma, J., & Schiedermayer, D. L. (1991). The bookie, the girlfriend and the vultures. *Annals of Internal Medicine, 151*, 98.

La Puma, J., & Schiedermayer, D. L. (1994). *Ethics consultation: A practical guide.* Boston: Jones and Bartlett.

Loewy, E. H. (1992). Advance directives and surrogate laws: Ethical instruments or moral cop-out? *Archives of Internal Medicine, 152*, 1973–1977.

Malloy, T. R., Wigton, R. S., Meeske, J., & Tape, T. G. (1992). The influ ence of treatment descriptions on advance medical directive decisions. *Journal of the American Geriatrics Society, 40,* 1255–1260.

Menikoff, J. A., Sachs, G. A., & Seigler, M. (1992). Beyond advance directives—health care surrogate laws. *New England Journal of Medicine, 327,* 1165–1169.

Moody, H. R. (1992). *Ethics in an aging society.* Baltimore: Johns Hopkins University Press.

Nash, D. (1994). *Managed care: A survival guide for the 90s.* Rockville, MD: Aspen.

Schneiderman, L. J., Pearlman, R. A., Kaplan, R. M., Anderson, J. P., & Rosenberg, E. M. (1992). Relationship of general advance directive instructions to specific life-sustaining treatment preferences in patients with serious illness. *Archives of Internal Medicine, 152,* 2114–2122.

Simpson, K. (1993). Health care surrogate laws. *New England Journal of Medicine, 328,* 1200.

Wagner, A. (1984). Cardiopulmonary resuscitation in the aged. *New England Journal of Medicine, 310*(17), 1129–1130.

Wetle, T., Levkoff, S., Cwikel, J., & Rosen, A. (1988). Nursing home resident participation in medical decisions: Perceptions and preferences. *Gerontologist, 28* (Suppl.), 32–38.

## THE CASE OF MS. A

Ms. F has been a resident in your nursing home for several years. Several weeks ago, she suffered a major stroke and has been in a coma ever since. Ms. F has no advance directives and, according to her family and her primary care team, had never discussed her treatment preferences. An IV is started, and after a few days, the IV is discontinued and a nasogastric tube is inserted for feeding.

Ms. F's roommate, Ms. A, is very distressed by Ms. F's condition. She sees Ms. F continue to receive treatment; she is bathed daily, turned and positioned every 2 hours, receives mouth care and nasogastric feedings. However, there is no response whatsoever from Ms. F.

Dr. Smith is responsible for the care of both Ms. A and Ms. F. One day, after Dr. Smith has visited Ms. F, Ms. A approaches him and asks how long he expects that Ms. F will go on in her condition. Dr. Smith replies that it is possible for Ms. F to survive for quite a long time, given her general condition and the fact that she is being maintained on tube feedings. Ms. A says she would never want to live like that. Dr. Smith asks Ms A if she would like to talk about what kinds of treatments she would or would not prefer to have if she were ever in a condition similar to Ms. F. Ms. A replies, "Oh, no—I don't want that responsibility!"

## QUESTIONS FOR DISCUSSION

1. What should Dr. Smith say to Ms. A?
2. Would there be any advantage to bringing more members of the primary health care team (e. g., the social worker, nurse, or nursing assistant) into the conversation? Why or why not?
3. How common do you think it is for nursing home residents to execute advance directives?
4. Should Ms. A's family be informed of the conversation between Dr. Smith and Ms. A and asked to communicate with Ms. A?
5. Should Dr. Smith ask Ms. A what she believes he should do about the case of Ms. F?

## ANSWERS

Dr. Smith must tread a very fine line between exploring Ms. A's feelings regarding her roommate's care and possibly her own and not coercing Ms. A to make statements or decisions with which she is not comfortable. As a matter of course, he should ask other members of the health care team if Ms. A has ever expressed wishes to them, and perhaps they would facilitate the discussion. If not, Dr. Smith must work to develop a relationship with Ms. A over time that fosters open communication and trust. If for any reason Dr. Smith feels that this is not possible or that time is too short and Ms. A is facing impending problems, he may turn to other members of the health care team who are closer to her to pursue discussion or may involve any close family member. However, if he chooses to speak to her family, he should discuss this with Ms. A prior to doing so.

Dr. Smith or other members of Ms. A's primary care team might ask Ms. A what it is about Ms. F's situation that distresses her before discussing in more detail what treatment(s) is most likely keeping her alive. It may be more helpful to Ms. A to reflect on her own feelings about quality of life, rather than on individual treatments that she might not fully understand or feel it is not her duty to know about. It is not certain what percentage of nursing home residents (or even people in general) have advance directives (Cassel & Zweibel, 1987; Emanuel & Emanuel, 1990; High, 1988), but if Ms. A never completed one, she would not be alone. In fact, she would clearly be in the majority. Some research has been conducted on impediments to completing advance directives, but it is still not clear why people do not complete them (La Puma, Orentlicher, & Moss, 1991; Sachs, Stocking, & Miles, 1992; Stetler, Elliott, & Bruno, 1992).

If after a few attempts at giving Ms. A an opportunity to discuss her feelings about quality of life and treatment preferences (if the discussions even go that far) she is still reluctant, her wish not to make a decision should be respected. She should at this time, however, be made aware of the possibility of appointing someone else to make decisions for her should she become mentally incapacitated. Many older people, especially those with family (Gamble, McDonald, & Lichstein, 1991; High, 1988), find this option preferable. If she is still reluctant, it should be left that any time she wishes to reopen the discussion, she should contact those people deemed to be the ones she would be most comfortable with discussing these matters. The physician and social worker should continue to visit regularly to facilitate this option.

If Ms. A was not included in the discussion of what Ms. F's wishes for treatment might have been, she should have been. Even though she is not family, Ms. F may have shared her thoughts with her regarding treatment preferences in certain situations and conditions under which she would not want to live.

## REFERENCES

Cassel, C. K. & Zweibel, N. R. (1987). Attitudes regarding life-extending medical care among the elderly and their children [Special issue]. *Gerontologist, 27,* 229A.

Emanuel, E. J. & Emanuel, L. L. (1990). Living wills: Past, present and future. *Journal of Clinical Ethics, 1*(1), 9–19.

Gamble, E. R., McDonald, P., & Lichstein, P. (1991). Knowledge, attitudes, and behavior of elderly patients regarding living wills. *Archives of Internal Medicine, 151*(2), 289–294.

High, D. M. (1988). All in the family: Extended autonomy and expectations in surrogate health care decision-making. *Gerontologist, 28*(Suppl.), 46–52.

La Puma, J., Orentlicher, D., & Moss, R. J. (1991). Advance directives on admission: Clinical implications and analysis of the Patient Self-Determination Act. *Journal of the American Medical Association, 266*(3), 402–405.

Sachs, G. A., Stocking, C. B., & Miles, S. H. (1992). Empowerment of the older patient? A randomized, controlled trial to increase discussion and use of advance directives. *Journal of the American Geriatrics Society, 40,* 269–273.

Stetler, K. L., Elliott, B. A., & Bruno, C. A. (1992). Living will completion in older adults. *Archives of Internal Medicine, 152,* 954–959.

# 2

# Multiculturalism in Nursing Homes

*Philip Boyle*

The increasing recognition of the plurality of cultural perspectives, the fact of "multiculturalism," is creating a number of ethical issues for nursing home administrators, ethicists, and ethics committees (Rankin & Kappy, 1993). As they attempt to accommodate cultural differences within their walls, they find themselves challenging institutional stability and long-cherished values. Everyone agrees that institutions such as nursing homes should respect differences of ethnicity, race, gender, and religion. Yet little agreement exists about how to respect and how far to go in respecting the particular identities of those who populate nursing homes, as well as those who work within the home.

An example of the potential conflict created by multiculturalism found in nursing homes is the tradition among certain cultures whereby families make health care decisions for even competent family members (Klessing, 1992). In a society that promotes autonomous decision making, is it possible to simultaneously balance the need to respect residents whose heritage favors family decision making and the need to protect deeply held U.S. values such as autonomous patient decision making? The desire to respect cultural differences can seemingly place prized values of the dominant culture in jeopardy. Consequently, one inadequate response is to ignore cultural differences altogether, on the plea that respecting those differences is too inefficient or will undercut established order in nursing home life. In contrast, a response that respects those differences creates an ethical head-ache over how extensive a nursing home's obligations are. Part of the dilemma is practical—dealing with the fact of multi-culturalism. Is there a clinically workable solution to cultural conflicts that does not diminish the values of minority cultures and simultaneously protects the cherished values of the domi-nant culture? Who will make the decision between clashing cul-tural values? Will the decision be perceived as coercive and anti-thetical to the commitments of the moral pluralists, or will it be the product of consensus and place at risk institutional values? Another part of the dilemma creates problems for ethical theory—dealing with a theory of plural values. Will respect for cultural difference foster an unhealthy moral relativism that practically might undercut institutional authority? How can society admit plural moral values, and by what means will it decide between seemingly irreconcilable values? Are cultural differences of equal or similar weight?

## RELIGIOUS MULTICULTURALISM: THE PLURALITY OF RELIGIONS CLASH

A full explanation of the challenges created by every kind of cul-tural difference is impossible in a limited space, but in long-term care one difference—religious—is more pronounced and an im-portant source of tension compared to acute care. However, les-sons learned from resolving conflicts involving religion can be extrapolated to other problematic areas of difference, such as race, socioeconomic background, and education.

In acute care, religious difference is seldom of significance, except in religiously sponsored institutions that forbid some kinds of treatment modalities. For example, Catholic-sponsored hospi-tals prohibit abortions, sterilizations, and in some cases, the with-drawal of nutrition and hydration from patients who are in a persistent vegetative state. The sheer amount of time that people spend in a long-term care facility—an average of approximately 3 years (USDHHS, 1989)—makes it more likely that the religious differences will become significant in the day-to-day life of both residents and staff.

It has been argued elsewhere (Collopy, Boyle, & Jennings, 1991) that the moral dilemmas in nursing homes should be examined in light of such questions as what kind of place do we want this home to be or what will bring human flourishing within this home? If religious sentiment has been part of a resident's flourishing before entering a home, then the home cannot simply ask people to leave religious faith at the door. To produce a moral environment that is productive of human flourishing, nursing homes must pay attention to conflicts that occur over religious differences. This will entail developing a more complex notion of how to balance the value issues generated by religious views (Lovin & Reynolds, 1992).

In resolving problems created by religious differences, anyone would be struck by the special twists these differences create. On the one hand, religious difference is for the most part easier to spot than other kinds of difference because it is usually created by readily identifiable doctrines. On the other hand, religious difference is more difficult to address and perhaps even convenient to ignore. Some people ignore it altogether because they think religious convictions are irrational, and it seems incomprehensible to them that one might structure life choices on doctrinal beliefs. Others set aside religious conflict as having no public standing in institutional settings, roughly the distinction between church and state. In a pluralistic society, in which we are uncertain about how to resolve religious claims, they are usually overlooked.

So how should nursing homes split the difference over religious conflicts? How much should religion matter, if at all? How far should we go in honoring or restricting religious difference? When should it be dominant over other important values?

## GERALDO, NO! DISNEY CHANNEL, NO!

In a nondenominational nursing home with a long waiting list for entrance, two roommates were in a battle over television viewing. One roommate watched television constantly in the bedroom because she was unable to watch her favorite shows on the home's community television. Her roommate was a moderately demented, extremely religious woman whose daughter and two grandchildren would visit every afternoon for 3 hours. The daughter regularly complained that the soap operas, talk shows, and in fact, any programming were morally offensive to her mother, herself, and especially her children. She demanded that the television be turned off during her daily visit, but the roommate protested that she would then miss her favorite shows.

Attempts to come to a workable solution seemed at a standstill. A dominant position among the staff was that because the very religious resident remained cognitively impaired, she was unaffected by the programs her daughter judged offensive. In fact, the staff observed the religious resident laughing, maybe enjoying the programming because the noise and motion were stimulating her. Moreover, the staff claimed that their primary obligation was to the resident, not the resident's family. The religious wishes of the daughter should have no standing. For most staff the issue was not a philosophical problem of how to honor religious sensitivities but an administrative problem that aimed at minimizing conflict. It is reasonable to ask, therefore, what one actually gains by sensitivity to religious diversity in resolving this conflict.

To understand the impact of a sensitivity to religious difference, it would first be important to examine the case from a perspective devoid of religious sensitivities. An ethics committee might frame the problem, for example, as one determining how logistically difficult it would be for the staff to accommodate the different parties. They might investigate the privileges and responsibilities of all of the parties involved. The resident who watches TV certainly seems entitled to be in her room and pursue activities that do not create a physical hazard for the roommate. The very pious roommate, no matter how demented, has a claim to have her wishes respected as long as some sense of those can be gathered. Simple fairness—doing unto others as you would have them do unto you—would be a reason for the television-watching roommate to respect the wishes of the demented woman if they were known, but they are not. Possibly, the woman in her present demented state was being stimulated by the noise and motion of the programming. In an analysis devoid of religious sensitivity, the investigation might have concluded at this point that it was all right for the television to be on. However, the daughter, who is the legal agent of the demented resident, has an obligation to promote her mother's wishes and best interests. Even though her mother's wishes about particular programming are not known, the daughter claims that the mother's lifelong piety suggests that she would object to the television programming if she were in a position to do so. An analysis of this case without religious sensitivity would at this point conclude that both sides have equal claims and that there is no way out of the impasse.

If religious difference were taken into account, the analysis would go otherwise. Although it is unclear how much the demented woman benefits from the daily family visits, they do create a situation that to some extent approximates her life before she entered the nursing home. Her previous life was one filled with piety and observance of religious custom. Her connection to that past is her daughter's ability to maintain that observance on her behalf. An analysis that assumes that nursing homes are not places to go to die, but rather places where human lives can be lived out meaningfully even in the twilight of one's life, would require added attempts to respect the demented woman's religious past. Whereas an analysis unobservant of religious views might lead to a standoff about what is required, a contrasting view that is sensitive to religious difference would require more action if nursing homes are to become places for human fulfillment.

So what would be gained from trying to split the religious difference? First, it demonstrates that paying attention to cultural differences, including religious ones, is a "way of seeing." It enables those who are doing an ethical analysis to note human values that might otherwise be overlooked. Second, it shows that there is no easy way to weight plural values (Kekes, 1993; Taylor, 1992). It is not at all obvious that the value of watching the TV is greater or lesser than the value of protecting religious sensitivities. As a practical outcome, those attempting to analyze the conflict, for example, might see the alternative as finding these residents new roommates with compatible religious sensitivities and in the future to making certain that upon admission roommates are paired not only on the basis of religion but also on the degree to which they have observed their religion—how faithfully they have adhered to its customs and practices in the past.

## RELIGIOUS DIVERSITY AND SEXUAL RELATIONS

In a nonsectarian nursing home two nurses encountered two residents in a public lounge in the beginning stages of sexual intercourse. They pulled the couple apart. Considerable disagreement arose among staff members about how to respond to the incident between the male resident, whose wife visited regularly with their grandchildren, and the never-married female resident, who had a history of mental disorders and sexually active behavior. Many options were discussed. Should the nursing home permit sexual behavior between any consenting residents or limit the activity to married residents? Would the staff be sanctioning marital infidelity if they let this male resident continue? Should the staff attempt to curb his activity with threats to tell his wife? If they permit sexual activity, are they obligated to provide a separate space for such activity so as to avoid a possible disturbance between roommates?

At first blush the issue of religious diversity was absent from the discussion. Yet all of the questions seem to hinge on how to resolve one fundamental issue: sexual relations outside marriage. It became evident to the committee that most staff members were objecting to the behavior based on a religious perspective— religion with a lowercase *r*. Their objections were based not on any clearly identifiable religious doctrine but on cultural norms that are deeply held and believed. Only a minority of staff members objected on the basis of a religious doctrine of their church. The ethics committee was faced with the problem of which view— that of the prevailing culture, shared by the staff, or that of the couple—should prevail. If the home had a religious sponsor with a clearly articulated prohibition against such activity, the staff would have plain direction. But as it was, the conflict was between different religious conceptions—both with a lowercase *r*— of what was acceptable behavior.

A serious exploration of religious difference would naturally confront several issues. Clearly, there is no obviously greater or lesser weight for either of the conflicting values. One quick way to resolve this standoff is simply to encourage toleration when religious conflicts arise. However, this short-circuiting of moral investigation will not produce as reliable a set of conclusions as will a thorough moral analysis.

As in any useful ethics evaluation, it is important to identify areas of agreement and disagreement. For example, everyone agreed that the couple should not show sexual affection in public places, where it would be offensive, and that the public lounge should be treated like any other public space where such activity would be prohibited. After exhausting this line of investigation, it might become apparent that the primary locus of disagreement was over private sexual relations between residents. However, even after the locus of conflict is framed, a clear decision might not be available.

Although no benefit of further analysis seems obvious, there is at least one for those who investigate the conflict. To pay attention to the particularities is to bring a fuller meaning to ethics: it is a realization that the act of moral struggle makes us more human. Only by paying attention to all of the subtleties through sensitive moral analysis do we fully honor others and become more fully human ourselves (Nussbaum, 1990).

Another benefit for wading deeply into religious difference is an understanding of how decisions over plural values get made. This first reaction to the couple by the staff—and the common one at the home—shows that decisions about plural values were decided by those in authority and with the power to enforce it. Negotiation was absent. Those who would be affected most by the decision did not participate in it. It is a stance that inherently denies the possibility of plural values. Only a process that not only sees that there are plural values but also realizes that the resolution of conflicts among them cannot be simply by the exertion of power—something akin to a hegemony—is one that is consistent with a theory of plural values.

A final benefit is a better understanding of present and future options available for the ethics committee and the staff. For example, if residents were in a situation where they had the means and opportunity to choose long-term care that fit their values nicely, then the burden of a nursing home to be "all things to all people" would be lessened. Due to bed shortages in the region, both residents had been forced into this home as the only option. Obligations to toleration might be lessened if options were available to the parties involved. Deeper analysis might have also shown that for the future and beyond the issue of adultery, it would be wise to address the issue of whether there should be policies about sex in general. Policy is probably needed on the issue of whether the facility should afford residents the opportunity to express their sexuality in private.

## RELIGIOUS DIVERSITY AND WITHHOLDING LIFE-SUSTAINING TREATMENT

An 86-year-old Protestant woman residing in a Catholic nursing home was eating less and less due to stomach pain. The dietitian and nurse's aides insisted that she was trying to kill herself by refusing to eat, and they tried to force her to do so. They claimed that Catholic teaching forbids Catholic institutions to allow patients to forgo all nutrition and hydration, which would result in death. The woman's family maintained that she was fully capacitated and that if she refused to eat she should not be force-fed. As the family became more agitated over the force-feeding they began to talk down to the staff, who in turn responded combatively. The ethics committee was called for a consultation.

As in the previous case, it might seem that paying attention to religious difference is useless. From one perspective, religious views should have no bearing whatsoever. Capacitated people are constitutionally guaranteed the right to direct their medical care, even if this includes refusing care, and by refusing might end in the person's death. From another perspective, the fact that the home is sponsored by the Catholic church overrides any other religious or cultural perspective of residents and staff. According to this perspective, in order to maintain its religious identity, a home can restrict practices that are inconsistent with its doctrine. It does not have to honor values that are inconsistent with its beliefs but must simply inform the resident upon admission of the institutional stance. Because the home had not informed the resident upon admission, many staff members thought the dispute was an open-and-shut case—honor the woman's wishes this time but make provision for new residents by informing them upon admission that they will be force-fed if they refuse to eat. Neither perspective admits any room for negotiation; religious views are useless from the first perspective and dominant in the second. So what would an ethics committee gain from further sensitivity and exploration of religious difference?

In this case a religious sensitivity would have first required being clear about the scope, meaning, and authority of the religious teaching. For example, what is the exact Catholic teaching on withholding or withdrawing nutrition and hydration? By what authority was it taught—by a pope, by all bishops or just some, or only by theologians? For how long has it been taught—is it a recent statement or an ancient teaching? And under what circumstances was it taught—was it directed toward people in this resident's circumstances? Such an investigation would have shown that the dietitians and nurse's aides were unclear about the scope, meaning, and authority of the religious teaching. Formal teaching about nutrition and hydration is relatively new, beginning within the past decade, and at that it has been limited to a small number of U.S. bishops (U.S. Bishops, 1992). These bishops state that there should be a presumption in favor of providing nutrition and hydration for patients in a persistent vegetative state. An ethics committee that decided to be more sensitive to religious issues would have found that the authority of the teaching is weak because it is new and claimed by only a few bishops. Thus, religious sensitivity would have shown those who objected that they needed to know more about their own claims.

This posture of openness requires full examination of the weight of the clashing values. Examination at times can demonstrate that the value at stake is misunderstood or that it does not have the force it was first perceived to possess. Also, it can demonstrate that even within subgroups there is diversity; subgroups are not monoliths but often contain a rich assortment of views.

## CONCLUSIONS

So how do we balance the religious conflicts in nursing homes? First, whoever is doing the analysis will benefit from identifying values that are often run over roughshod.

Second, it is important to realize that sensitivity to religious diversity does not necessarily require that cherished values be disposed of. Many aspects of the religious difference must be examined and weighed before any conclusion is warranted. Is the difference clearly identified? Does the difference arise from explicit religious doctrine, or does it arise out of misinterpretation or an interpretation of the strength or weakness of religious doctrine? No one would be required to be sensitive to differences that arise out of confusion of teaching or practice. But if the doctrine is clear, then there must be an analysis of whether the doctrine is central to the identity of the institution. For example, is the nursing home sponsored by a religious organization? If, on the other hand, the difference is between individual residents or between a nonsectarian home and a resident, religious conflict will need to be weighed against other important values.

Third, some attempts to resolve the difference will be impossible. Theories of moral plural values that wrestle with the fact and conflicts of multiculturalism fully acknowledge that in some cases no conclusive result will be possible. Whether the clash of values is created by religion, ethnicity, race, or gender, the incommensurability of the values will lead to an impasse at times. Nonetheless, the process of moral struggle is not merely to arrive at a clinical solution. Those who struggle to split the difference honor others and in doing so become more human.

## REFERENCES

Collopy, B., Boyle, P., & Jennings, B. (1991, March–April). New directions in nursing home ethics. *The Hastings Center Report* (Special Suppl.), 1–15.

Kekes, J. (1993). The morality of pluralism. Princeton, NJ: Princeton University Press.

Klessing, J. (1992). Cross-cultural medicine a decade later: The effect of values and culture on life-support decisions. *The Western Journal of Medicine, 157* (3), 316–322.

Lovin, R., & Reynolds, R. (1992). Focus: Ethical naturalism and indigenous cultures. *Journal of Religious Ethics, 20,* 267–415.

Nussbaum, M. (1990). *Love's knowledge: Essays on philosophy and literature.* New York: Oxford University Press.

Rankin, S., & Kappy, M. (1993). Developing therapeutic relationships in multicultural settings. *Academic Medicine, 68,* 826–827.

Taylor, C. (1992). *Multiculturalism and the "politics of recognition."* Princeton, NJ: Princeton University Press.

U.S. Bishops' Pro-Life Committee. (1992). Nutrition and hydration: Moral and pastoral reflection. *Origins,* 705–712.

U.S. Department of Health and Human Services, Public Health Service. (1989). The national nursing home survey: 1985 summary for the United States: Data from the National Health survey. *Vital and Health Statistics,* Ser. 13, No. 9, (DHHS Publication No. PHS 89-1758). Washington, DC: U.S. Government Printing Office.

## THE CASE OF MS. B

Ms. B is an 80-year-old woman who has resided in your nursing home for 2 years. As the result of a disabling childhood illness, Ms. B has numerous functional limitations, although she is cognitively intact. Ms. B entered your facility very reluctantly when her physical disabilities increased to the extent that she could not function at home, even with the services of a home health aide.

Ms. B has two children, both daughters, who visit occasionally. Very active in politics and the arts in her community, Ms. B had many social contacts prior to admission. However, many of them have died, and most of her surviving friends are themselves quite physically frail. As a result, few of them are able to visit her now. When you speak with her, she mentions the "old days" with great nostalgia. Further, in addition to mourning the loss of many friends and social contacts, it is obvious to you when you speak with her that Ms. B is still grieving over the death of her husband, who died more than 5 years ago. Because your nursing home has a high proportion of residents with dementing illnesses, the pool from which Ms. B can draw new friends is limited.

Ms. B spends the majority of her time making demands of the staff on the floor where she resides. Although some of her demands are clearly legitimate, many of them seem inappropriate and unnecessary. The staff, whose workload is already quite heavy, is somewhat resentful of her constant demands. Without exception, all of the members of the primary care team responsible for her care find Ms. B difficult to please. Particularly problematic, however, are the interpersonal relationships between Ms. B and the nursing assistants. Many of the paraprofessional staff are members of ethnic minorities, who think Ms. B looks down on them. From her perspective, Ms. B believes the staff doesn't like her and that most of them regard her as a "spoiled rich old lady." She is also very resentful of the power they hold over her as she is dependent on them for assistance.

## QUESTIONS FOR DISCUSSION

1. What approach would you take with Ms. B?

2. What approach would you take with the team responsible for
Ms. B's care?


**ANSWERS**

This is one of the more difficult issues of institutional life, and
probably occurs with relative frequency given the degree of cultural diversity in nursing homes (Foldes, 1990). However, as with
other dilemmas, information gathering is one of the first steps.
Ms. B's feelings toward the staff must be explored in detail. In
the past, has she had similar problems with caregivers or with
people in general? It may be that Ms. B's personality is such that
you will not be able to change her behavior, as it is part of a long-
standing personality style. It may be helpful to ask social service
to assist in exploring this issue and to ask Ms. B if she would
mind if her family was involved in the discussion of the problems
she is having in the home. How much you should involve them
without her permission depends on her degree of mental capacity and how much understanding she has of her behavior. Although it might be possible to learn much from information obtained without her permission, doing so is probably suspect at
best with regard to what is ethical behavior in this situation on
the part of the staff. If it is determined that Ms. B is willing to
work with you to improve things, the staff should then be ap-
proached in a separate setting, informed of Ms. B's complaints,
and allowed to respond. Staff feelings and experiences regarding
the people they care for need to be explored, and what it means
to someone to enter institutional life, with all of its attendant
losses as well as benefits, should be reviewed with them. Ms. B
similarly needs to be educated as to the pressures and stigmata
that the nursing assistants in particular may feel are a part of
their job and encouraged to understand why they may react to
her the way they do.

   A contributing factor to Ms. B's behavior may clearly be bore-
dom, and she should be encouraged to channel her energies into
more positive behaviors. Also, her lack of social contacts may
have more to do with her behavior than the inadequate opportunities to interact with alert people in the nursing home setting.
About 50% of nursing home residents are estimated to be mentally intact (Ouslander, Osterweil, & Morley, 1991).

Ms. B should be evaluated medically to see if her condition(s) can be better treated to make her more comfortable and less complaining and whether she is suffering any untoward side effects of medication. The issue of apparent unresolved grief over the death of her husband should also be addressed by the staff.

## REFERENCES

Foldes, S. S. (1990). Life in an institution: A sociological and anthropological view. In R. A. Kane & A. L. Caplan (Eds.), *Everyday ethics: Resolving dilemmas in nursing home life*. New York: Springer Publishing Co.
Ouslander, J. G., Osterweil, D., & Morley, J. (1991). *Medical care in the nursing home*. New York: McGraw-Hill.

# 3

# Treatment Termination in Long-Term Care: Implications for Heatlh Care Providers

*Eileen R. Chichin*

Long-term care institutions are currently populated by increasing numbers of frail elderly suffering from dementing illnesses. This, in concert with a new awareness of patients' rights with respect to treatment decisions, has resulted in a rise in the numbers of requests to terminate life-prolonging treatment in nursing homes. Treatment termination clearly has profound implications for the individual who chooses this option, and of course, family members are also markedly affected. But what of the caregiving staff in nursing homes? How do requests to limit treatment and, more important, the deaths of residents as a result of treatment termination, impact upon the professionals and paraprofessionals who care for these residents?

Literature on grief and bereavement among health care providers who regularly care for dying patients suggests that these caregivers frequently experience grief reactions (Benoliel, 1974; Lerea & LiMauro, 1982; Lev, 1989), and the emotional difficulties associated with caring for the dying have been noted by many (Harper, 1977; Kastenbaum, 1967; Koocher, 1979; Rando, 1984; Strauss, 1968). However, there appears to be no empirical evidence of the effects on long-term care staff of caring for residents who die as a result of the termination of life-sustaining treatment. Anecdotal evidence suggests that, due to the intense and long-term relationships that develop between staff and residents, nursing home staff members often feel as if they are the surrogate family of the residents for whom they care. Surely, then, the death of any resident will impact upon the staff. And, one might assume, a death that ensues after treatment is terminated might be particularly painful for staff because treatment termination is often perceived by health care providers as counter to their training and philosophy. When treatment termination is involved, they who are so passionately involved in the preservation of life now see themselves as "causing" death.

In order to explore this further, to develop interventions to support the staff involved in caring for residents after treatment termination, and to assess the work of the ethics consult team at the Jewish Home and Hospital for Aged of New York,[1] the home's Center on Ethics began to follow up staff members whose residents died after life-prolonging treatment was withheld or withdrawn. What follows are some of the results of interviews with 15 staff members who cared for such residents. We feel these data offer some important initial insights into the effects on staff of caring for residents during treatment termination.

## INTERVIEW METHODS AND RESULTS

Using a questionnaire developed to study the impact of treatment termination on staff, interviews were conducted by research assistants in the Jewish Home's Center on Ethics. The 15 staff members interviewed represented a variety of disciplines, including nursing, social work, recreation therapy, and medicine. Three of the subjects were certified nursing assistants. All staff members had been employed in long-term care for varying periods but all for more than 1 year.

It should be noted that, in all cases at the time a particular life-prolonging treatment was withheld or withdrawn, none of the residents involved was capable of making a treatment decision. Therefore, treatment was terminated based on the previously expressed wishes of the resident. These wishes would have been made known through a living will, health care proxy, or some other source that was felt to meet New York State's stringent "clear and convincing evidence" standard.[2] In most cases in which there was no advance directive, clear and convincing evidence consisted of specific statements made over time by the resident when he or she was able to express preferences about a particular treatment.

The interview began with some forced-choice items assessing subjects' general feelings about working with dying patients and particularly about residents dying as a result of treatment termination. Answers to these items varied, depending upon the particular issue. For example, in response to the statement "Caring for a person who is dying is always emotionally draining," almost all staff members agreed. In contrast, subjects were more evenly divided on the issue "Caring for a person who is dying is a very satisfying experience, even if death is the result of withholding or withdrawing treatment." Two-thirds of the staff members interviewed said they felt that caring for a person who is dying from a disease over which they have no control is very different from caring for someone who dies because he or she requested that treatment be terminated.

Some of the literature on working with the dying suggests that this work engenders certain emotions in caregivers. Extrapolating from that work (see, e.g., Benoliel, 1974; Epstein, 1975), subjects in this study were asked if they experienced certain emotions as a result of caring for residents who died after treatment was withheld or withdrawn. Among these emotions were a sense of powerlessness, loss of composure, loss of control, loss of competence, and a sense of feeling stressed.

Interestingly, the only emotion that all staff members reported was the sense of feeling stressed. However, most of the subjects reported a sense of powerlessness, and only two said they never felt a loss of control.

Staff members were then asked a number of questions about their experience with a particular resident. Because the quality of the relationship between the staff member and the resident was thought to influence the staff member's feelings about treatment termination, subjects were asked how close they felt to the resident and if the degree of closeness made caring for the resident easier or more difficult.

Most of the staff members who were interviewed said they felt either very close or somewhat close to the resident. Further, they said that this closeness made caring for the dying resident more difficult, often explaining that the resident had become like a family member to them. Some said they felt that it would have been easier to make treatment termination decisions for strangers, rather than for a person toward whom one felt close.

It was also believed that the degree of comfort that staff members had with the plan to withhold or withdraw life-sustaining treatment would influence their feelings. Therefore, the following question was asked: "When it was decided that the resident would not want life-prolonging treatment in his or her current situation, how satisfied were you that the right thing was being done?" In most cases, staff members said they were quite satisfied that the right thing was being done. When asked why, they were likely to cite three factors that contributed to their degree of comfort with treatment termination: the existence of clearly written evidence of the resident's wishes, a sense of being involved in the decision-making process, and extensive discussions between the resident's primary care team and the ethics consult team.

When asked just what it was about a resident's dying process that is most difficult for caregiving staff, most staff members' answers centered on watching the gradual deterioration of a resident to whom a staff member felt particularly close. Several responses also focused on the difficulties associated with trying to determine the resident's level of discomfort and the staff's frustration and ambivalence about the entire situation. The staff made statements such as "[The most difficult thing for me was] seeing the resident deteriorate so quickly and knowing that I was actively involved in this process" and "[What was difficult for me was] trying to determine whether she was having any discomfort and how to determine at what point she wasn't going to get any better." One social worker summed up the feelings of all of the staff involved in these cases when she said, "I just wish this didn't have to happen."

In trying to determine which particular aspects of this process were most difficult for the staff, subjects were asked: "Of all the things you were required to do for this resident while he or she was dying, what was the most difficult?" Responses here fell into two categories: the physical and the emotional. Included among the physical were the actual discontinuation of treatment (i.e., removing the nasogastric tube or discontinuing the IV)—what one staff member called "the final act." One nurse was particularly distressed by being asked by the family and the physician to administer pain medication when she felt that by so doing she "was pushing the patient over the edge."

Among the emotional issues that the staff cited as difficult were the provision of emotional support to the resident and also to the family. One social worker said that just sitting with the resident was most difficult for her. Nonetheless, although this evoked a profound sense of sadness in her, she continued to do it and also encouraged all primary care team members to take turns sitting with the resident.

Interestingly, staff members reported that the things that were most difficult for them while the resident was dying seemed also to provide the most satisfaction. They cited feeling especially good about providing good physical care—turning and positioning, wetting lips, giving sips of water, and administering adequate pain medication. They also felt good about the provision of emotional support, with touching the resident and holding the resident's hand cited most often, followed by talking to residents and telling them that the staff would do everything in their power to keep them comfortable. One nurse stated that she derived satisfaction from attempting to give oral fluids to the dying resident, bringing her flowers, and repeatedly telling her she would keep her as comfortable as possible.

The provision of emotional support to family and other staff members was also mentioned as making staff members feel especially good, with social workers in particular deriving satisfaction from supporting other staff. One social worker said: "I couldn't do anything for the resident because she was in a coma. However, I was able to support the nursing assistants and help them accept that Mrs. S's wishes might be different from their own."

To determine whether anything was helpful to staff members during this difficult process, subjects were asked: "While this resident was dying, was there anything anyone at the Home did that made the experience any easier for you, or that you found especially helpful?" Here, all of the responses fell into the category of emotional support, especially from colleagues and members of the ethics consult team. One social worker mentioned that her job of supporting the family was made easier because the physician on the ethics consult team made herself available by telephone to the family around the clock. This made family members feel that they were closely involved in the treatment plan and had some degree of control over the process.

It was anticipated that the difficulties associated with caring for a person during treatment termination would not end at the time of the resident's death. Therefore, staff members were asked what was helpful to them after the resident died. Again, not surprisingly, emotional support from a wide variety of individuals was cited time and time again. Of particular note, however, were the responses to the question "Was any one person especially helpful?" Responses here ranged from family and friends of staff members to clergy and to staff members within the institution, but members of the nursing department were very likely to mention the support of the director of nursing as the most helpful. Similarly, the social workers who participated in the study cited support of the director of social work as most helpful. This suggests that, although family, friend, and interdisciplinary emotional support is helpful, feeling supported by the administrative staff of one's own discipline is probably key to a staff member's comfort during this particularly difficult time.

## DISCUSSION AND IMPLICATIONS

Clearly apparent throughout all of these interviews is the emotional pain experienced by staff members caring for residents during treatment termination. As noted earlier, all staff members reported feeling stressed, and most said they took their worries and concerns about the case home with them. When a person has advanced dementia, as is the case in the majority of these treatment-termination situations, some think that he or she is not suffering. Rather, it is the survivors—the families, friends, and caregivers—who are suffering. Further compounding the psychic pain experienced by health care providers when they are involved in caring for someone who has opted to forgo life-sustaining treatment may be the perception that their work is meaningless. Is that the case when work one performed for months and years to keep a person alive is now intentionally stopped? It has been suggested (Lev, 1989) that perhaps the grief of health care providers is exacerbated when individuals "perceived to be without hope are being cared for" (p. 290). In addition, society in general and many health-related professions in particular place special emphasis on sustaining life. Nearly 20 years ago, Jeanne Quint Benoliel (1974) wrote:

> Given that the medical and nursing subcultures attach primary value to
> life-saving activity and secondary value to palliation and symptomatic

therapy, the performance of tasks associated with the preservation of life carries greater weight in the allocation of professional and social rewards than does the provision of comfort (p. 220).

Two decades later, her words still seem to ring somewhat true.

Given society's views on life prolongation, in concert with the socialization of many health care professionals toward a "cure" rather than a "care" orientation, caring for the caregiver involved in treatment termination is a formidable, although not insurmountable, task. Our experience to date suggests that the most important interventions fall into the category of emotional support of staff members. It is likely that many of the mechanisms identified in the literature on professionals working with frail elderly and in hospice settings are transferrable to health care providers involved in caring for patients dying after treatment termination. Peer support has been found to ameliorate symptoms of burnout in human service workers (Carrilio & Eisenberg, 1984). In addition, team interaction has been found to provide both physical and emotional support in hospice workers (Riordan & Salzer, 1992). Accordingly, both one-to-one and group interactions with supervisors, peers, and interdisciplinary team members should be utilized regularly by those caring for persons dying after life-sustaining treatment is withheld or withdrawn. All staff members need to be permitted to express their feelings about these difficult issues without fear of judgment (Lev, 1989).

Riordan and Salzer (1992), in summarizing the literature on burnout experienced by health care providers working with the terminally ill, suggest that those who do this kind of work can be helped by attention to four specific areas: physical, psychological, intellectual, and spiritual. Interventions in these areas might also be helpful to those involved in the difficult task of caring for patients who die as a result of treatment termination.

With respect to the physical, health care providers caring for those who are dying need to ensure that they get adequate rest and exercise and to be particularly careful to avoid the buildup of tension. Psychological interventions include such things as meditation, journal writing, and, when needed, professional therapy. Among the intellectual tasks that can be done to assist health care providers to ameliorate stress is keeping abreast of current writings in the field to maintain a sense of mastery. Given the paucity of literature to date specifically on the impact of treatment termination on caregiving staff, this might not be possible for these workers. However, related literature, for example articles dealing with comfort care in end-stage dementia, might prove helpful.

Two other areas that fall under intellectual interventions include an awareness of the need to increase interpersonal skills, and developing and maintaining a sense of humor. And finally, Riordan and Salzer's (1992) suggestions in the spiritual area include such things as engaging in traditional religious practices and enjoying the beauty of nature and the joys of friends and family.

We also need to constantly remind staff members that the greatest gift we can give to nursing home residents is respect for their wishes (Meyers, 1992) and to educate them in methods of making the dying process and death as comfortable and dignified as possible. Reinforcing to the staff the moral and legal rights of individuals to make treatment decisions, even when those decisions are at odds with the preferences of the professionals, may also be helpful.

In contrast to the ethicist Teo Forcht Dagi (1992), who contends that the needs of caregivers have no place in ethical decision making, it is suggested that to ignore these needs may be counterproductive if we expect these caregivers to implement such decisions. It is difficult to care for another if one's own needs and feelings are unrecognized. Yet unfortunately, implicit in the education of many health care professionals is the idea that to be "professional" one must rise above one's feelings, in essence denying that one is human. Better perhaps, for health care provider and patient alike, may be the recognition and acceptance of the professional's humanity—the understanding that to be a caring professional one must first be a caring human being. And if health care professionals and paraprofessionals are to be able to give of themselves, particularly in these most difficult cases involving treatment termination, they must also receive care and support.

## NOTES

1. See Olson, Chichin, Libow, Martico-Greenfield, Neufeld, and Mulvihill (1993) for a detailed description of the ethics consult team.
2. New York state, like Missouri, requires "clear and convincing" evidence of a person's wishes with regard to life-sustaining treatment before such treatment can be withheld or withdrawn.

## REFERENCES

Benoliel, J. Q. (1974). Anticipatory grief in physicians and nurses. In B. Schoenberg, A. C. Carr, A. H. Kutscher, D. Peretz, & I. K. Goldberg (Eds.), *Anticipatory grief.* New York: Columbia University Press.

Carrilio, T. E., & Eisenberg, D. M. (1984). Using peer support to prevent worker burnout. *Social Casework, 12,* 307–310.

Dagi, T. F. (1992). Compassion, consensus, and conflict: Should the caregivers' needs influence the ethical dialectic? *Journal of Clinical Ethics, 3*(3), 214–218.

Epstein, C. (1975). *Nursing the dying patient.* Reston, VA: Reston Publishing Co.

Harper, B. (1977). *Death: The coping mechanism of the health professional.* Greenville, SC: Southeastern University Press.

Kastenbaum, R. (1967). Multiple perspectives on a geriatric "Death Valley." *Community Mental Health Journal 3,* 21–29.

Koocher, G. (1979). Adjustment and coping strategies among the caretakers of cancer patients. *Social Work in Health Care, 5,* 145–151.

Lerea, L. E. & LiMauro, B. F. (1982). Grief among health care workers: A comparative study. *Journal of Gerontology, 37*(5), 604–608.

Lev, E. (1989). A nurse's perspective on disenfranchised grief. In K. Doka (Ed.), *Disenfranchised grief.* Lexington, MA: D. C. Heath.

Meyers, H. (1992, November). *The administrator's role.* Paper presented at a symposium on early experiences of ethics rounds and an ethics consult team. 45th Annual Scientific Meeting of the Gerontological Society of America, Washington, DC.

Olson, E., Chichin, E. R., Libow, L. S., Martico-Greenfield, T., Neufeld, R. R., & Mulvihill, M. (1993). A center on ethics in long-term care. *Gerontologist 33* (2), 269-274.

Olson, E., Chichin, E., Meyers, H., Schulman, E., & Brennan, F. (1994). Early experiences of an ethics consult team. *Journal of the American Geriatrics Society 42* (4), 363–463.

Rando, T. (1984). *Grief, dying and death: Clinical interventions for caregivers.* Champaign, IL: Research Press.

Riordan, R. J., & Salzer, S. K. (1992). Burnout prevention among health care providers working with the terminally ill: A literature review. *Omega, 25*(1), 17–24.

Strauss, A. (1968). The intensive care unit: Its characteristics and social relationships. *Nursing Clinics of North America, 3,* 7–15.

## THE CASE OF MS. C

Ms. C is a 95-year-old woman who was admitted to your nursing home nearly 2 years ago after suffering a right-sided CVA with left-sided hemiplegia. The stroke left her with some physical limitations, but she was cognitively intact. Shortly after admission, Ms. C's lawyer, who had known her for several years, visited her and assisted her in executing a living will. In that document, she stated that if she suffered from a condition in which there was "no reasonable expectation of recovery from physical or mental disability, I request that I be allowed to die and not be kept alive by artificial means or 'heroic measures.'" The types of treatments Ms. C mentioned specifically included "electrical or mechanical resuscitation of the heart when it has stopped beating, mechanical respiration by machine when the brain can no longer sustain breathing, nasogastric tube feedings when paralyzed or no longer able to swallow, and any invasive test or treatment."

Ms. C's only living relative was a cousin who visited regularly. However, she developed many close relationships with members of the primary care team responsible for her care.

Ms. C's primary care team noticed that she was slowly losing weight and had experienced a 12-lb. weight loss over a period of 5 months, from 115 to 103 lbs. They also noticed that she seemed to have trouble eating. After conducting a swallowing evaluation, the speech pathologist said that Ms. C had severe swallowing problems and strongly recommended that she not be fed by mouth, although she might be able to tolerate small feedings of sweet, thick substances. She could not, however, take in enough to sustain herself. This inability to swallow was felt to be an irreversible condition, and it was suspected that possibly Ms. C had suffered a second stroke. She also stopped talking, and it was unclear whether she was aphasic, depressed, angry, or in some other noncommunicative state.

Attempts were made to determine if Ms. C could give some indication of her wishes in this situation. However, she was unable or unwilling to answer questions, responding only "okay" when asked how she felt. Given that Ms. C seemed to meet a criterion mentioned in her living will ("when I am no longer able to swallow"), it was believed that she would not want to have a feeding tube inserted.

When you met with the primary care team responsible for Ms. C's care, you discussed with them her wishes as expressed in the living will. Members of the team, most of whom had grown very close to Ms. C, had never discussed artificial nutrition or hydration with her. However, they were reluctant not to insert a feeding tube, even after reading the living will. The nurses and nursing assistants in particular were concerned about not feeding someone who could still respond to them and would still accept food orally. The social worker, despite the fact that she had been present when Ms. C signed her living will, felt unsure about Ms. C's attitude toward tube feedings. However, when Ms. C's lawyer was contacted to see if he might know what Ms. C meant when she signed the living will, he said he felt she would not want a tube if her condition was indeed irreversible.

Because of lingering uncertainty about Ms. C's treatment wishes at this point in time and the irreversibility of her conditions, her primary care team and her lawyer agreed that a nasogastric feeding tube would be inserted as a temporary measure. However, Ms. C resisted very strongly any attempts to insert a tube. A gastrostomy tube was considered but was technically not possible due to a preexisting colostomy. Also, it was most likely inconsistent with her wishes for "no invasive treatment." Accordingly, she was given small amounts of her favorite food or fluid as tolerated, along with other comfort measures.

## QUESTIONS FOR DISCUSSION

1. Why was it important to determine that Ms. C's condition was irreversible?
2. What was the rationale behind attempting to determine treatment preferences directly from Ms. C?
3. Why was Ms. C's lawyer asked his opinion about Ms. C's intentions when making out the living will?
4. How appropriate was it for the primary care team to want to insert a feeding tube?
5. Should the feelings of the primary care team be taken into consideration when developing a treatment plan for Ms. C?
6. Could Ms. C's resistance to the insertion of the feeding tube be interpreted as a conscious refusal of this treatment?

7. Was it appropriate to consider a gastrostomy tube?
8. Is considering a feeding tube a "temporary" measure within accepted medical and ethical practice?

## ANSWERS

Many exceedingly frail older people may lose the ability or the desire to eat for reasons that are reversible, such as pneumonia or urinary tract infections. If properly diagnosed and treated, these conditions often resolve, and the older individual is again able to eat. Accordingly, before you consider implementing Ms. C's living will, it is important to ascertain the cause of her condition and to be convinced that it indeed cannot be treated and reversed. In addition, in order to respect her autonomy, it is important to determine whether, at this point in time, Ms. C can tell you her wishes regarding a tube feeding. All too often, frail older people with impaired decision-making ability are assumed to be unable to communicate their wishes. However, these individuals are often able to tell us what they would want, albeit often in simple terms, with regard to life-sustaining treatment. Further, it is important at least to consider that the treatment preferences delineated earlier in her living will may have changed as her circumstances changed. It has been suggested, for example, that persons in some stages of Alzheimer's disease may be quite content and comfortable, not experiencing the nightmare that many assume characterizes this disease. If this is so, they may want to amend their previously expressed treatment preferences (Drickamer & Lachs, 1992).

Another problem inherent in living wills is the inability of these documents to anticipate every eventuality that might befall us. Further, many of these documents, especially those executed several years ago, lack specificity, using, for example, terms such as "heroic measures" to describe treatments. In the case of Ms. C, even though her living will had been executed relatively recently, its wording was ambiguous and used the rather anachronistic term "heroic measures." Accordingly, the primary care team responsible for her care was unsure as to her intentions when she had the document drawn up. In these situations, it is often helpful to contact the individuals who witnessed the living will to determine if they were aware of the individual's intentions regarding treatment.

As long as the reversibility is *legitimately* in question, it is not inappropriate to provide adequate nutrition and hydration, even with means such as a nasogastric tube if necessary. In some cases, the reversibility of a condition could hinge on maintaining adequate nutrition.

Yet another issue that regularly surfaces in the long-term care setting is that of the relationships that develop between nursing home residents and their caregivers. Often, these relationships become so close that staff members become surrogate family to the residents for whom they care. Although some have argued that the feelings of caregivers should not influence treatment decisions, (see Dagi, 1992), failure to recognize these feelings can have deleterious effects on nursing home staff. In addition, many health care providers who accept a patient's right to refuse life-sustaining treatment on an intellectual level have great difficulty on an emotional level. This is even more difficult when communication with a patient is essentially impossible. Therefore, all staff members, including physicians, nurses, social workers, and nursing assistants, need to be supported as they carry out a nursing home resident's wishes to have life-sustaining treatment withheld or withdrawn and educated regarding residents' rights with respect to treatment termination.

Another intervention that can potentially benefit both the resident and the staff is a time-limited trial of treatment. In some situations, this will improve the resident's condition. However, even in those cases where no improvement is noted, the staff has the comfort of realizing they have tried every possible intervention. In addition, the passage of time may give staff members time to work through their feelings about the resident's decision.

In the case of Ms. C, as noted, all attempts to insert a nasogastric tube were unsuccessful. Some staff members may interpret this as a conscious attempt by Ms. C to make her wishes known. Although there is truly no way to make this determination, a cognitively impaired resident's resistance to this procedure sometimes suggests to staff that he or she does not want a feeding tube.

As far as inserting a gastrostomy tube is concerned, Ms. C's living will specifically stated she wanted no invasive procedures. This would clearly preclude the procedure necessary to insert the G-tube. However, had she not made that stipulation, it would also be acceptable to insert a G-tube as a time-limited trial. Although it is recognized that it is often far more difficult, on an emotional level, for health care providers to withdraw a treatment than it is to withhold the same treatment, most ethicists agree that there is no moral or ethical difference (Hastings Center, 1987). There is also legal support for this concept (Beauchamp & Childress, 1989; NY State Task Force, 1992). And from a medical standpoint, as noted above, providing artificial feeding for a time-limited period, whether by nasogastric or gastrostomy tube, may give a patient a chance for recovery he or she would not otherwise have had if no treatment was ever initiated.

## REFERENCES

Beauchamp, T. L., & Childress, J. F. (1989). *Principles of biomedical ethics* (3rd ed.). New York: Oxford University Press.

Dagi, T. F. (1992). Compassion, consensus, and conflict: Should the care givers' needs influence the ethical dialectic? *Journal of Clinical Ethics, 3*(3), 214–218.

Drickamer, M. A., & Lachs, M. S. (1992). Should patients with Alzheimer's disease be told their diagnosis? *New England Journal of Medicine, 326*(14), 947–951.

Hastings Center. (1987). *Guidelines on the termination of life-sustaining treatment and care of the dying.* Indianapolis: Indiana University Press.

New York State Task Force on Life and the Law. (1992). *When others must decide: Deciding for patients without capacity.* New York: Author.

# 4

# Treatment Termination in Long-Term Care: What about the Physician? What about the Family?

*Ellen Olson*

Despite what may be popular opinion, death has been a little-discussed issue in the nursing home. Most efforts in staff development are directed toward enhancing care and quality of life in the nursing home setting. Regulatory pressures are generally skewed toward aggressive care. Charts of both living and deceased residents are carefully scrutinized for any limitations or omissions in care that may be construed as patient abuse or neglect. Even though the legal climate in the nursing home has softened a bit, with increasing recognition and legitimization of advance directives and family decision making, the spector of regulatory scrutiny continues to limit or at least constrain the discussions of and possibilities for anything other than aggressive medical care in the nursing home. This phenomenon is not all necessarily driven by regulations, however. Many health care providers in the nursing home setting are conflicted about their own views on life and death and are uncomfortable with discussing limiting treatments, regardless of outside pressures. Many family members also, from a variety of other motivations, are not ready to let go of their elderly relative even in the most hopeless of situations and feed into the notion that only aggressive care will do, further confusing the health care provider as to the proper course of action.

The following questions should be asked: under what circumstances is it appropriate to consider limiting treatment in the nursing home, and does limiting treatment undermine both staff morale and public perceptions of nursing home care to a dangerous degree? Society has already answered the first question in that most, if not all, surveys of older persons and their end-of-life treatment decisions show that many would not want aggressive medical care if they were mentally incapacitated or terminally ill (Cohen-Mansfield et al., 1991; Emanuel, Barry, Stoeckle, Ettelson, & Emanuel, 1991; Lo, McCleod & Saika, 1986), conditions that describe a significant number of nursing home residents. As these wishes become more known through greater use and legal recognition of advance directives, health care providers must be prepared to honor these wishes and to work with families to ensure that their elderly incapacitated relatives are being cared for in a manner most consistent with their wishes.

Many physicians are clearly troubled by the trend toward limiting treatment in certain individuals, whether it is the patient himself or herself who refuses treatment or it is done through a surrogate decision maker. This phenomenon extends beyond the nursing home to all practice settings, except perhaps hospices. Although some physicians may limit treatments in older patients in particular, with too little consideration for patient or family preferences—and this phenomenon presents its own set of problems and solutions—the situation that confounds treatment decisions at the end of life most often is physician resistance to limiting treatment, especially when it involves those without the capacity to speak for themselves. An underlying motivation for this resistance may be what is perceived to be the increasing loss of physician autonomy. Through growing public awareness of patient autonomy, changes in and threats to reimbursement, and more complicated and stringent quality assurance practices, physicians are no longer left to their own devices in the practice of medicine.

This sense of loss may be further complicated in the nursing home setting, where the team approach has become the norm and the physician makes very few unilateral decisions, while still remaining accountable for all aspects of care. Medical treatment decisions may be the only area where the physician receives little

input from other team members and where professional autonomy may still prevail. Intrusion from staff or family may not be
welcomed. But even beyond that, there appears to be another
dynamic responsible for the discomfort that is inherent to the
medical profession and society in general, and that is a denial of
death as a reasonable outcome of care. This is not a new problem. In 1959, August Kaspar wrote:

> The average American's outlook on death seems to have changed some-
> time during the first quarter of the twentieth century. With great opti-
> mism, we embraced science and reason. Sin went out the window, and
> with it, its wages–death. Sickness became preventable and curable, and
> its companion, death, seemed equally vulnerable to our attack, an attack
> which was largely an elaborate denial of death. (p. 259)

He goes on to say that this changed the public perception of and
respect for physicians and allowed the physician to avoid the
thought of death if he or she wished to, saying that patients were
rarely rude enough to ask about it any more (Kasper, 1959).

Despite the subsequent hospice movement and books like
Kubler-Ross's (1969) *On Death and Dying*, the medical literature
continues to reflect the physician's preoccupation with life rather
than death, often citing Hippocrates and his strong stand against
physician-assisted death as the root of a professional obligation
to thwart death at all costs. Only in the past decade or so have
death and Hippocrates been reexamined. A letter to the editor
in the *Annals of Internal Medicine* regarding the Nancy Cruzan
case, written in support of family decision making versus that of
a court-appointed or bureaucratic system, states: "As technology
continues to advance, and we continue to keep patients 'alive,'
we physicians must learn to distinguish that line which separates
that which is done *for* a patient and that which is done *to* a patient" (p. 234). The author goes on to say that Hippocrates defined medicine in the following way:

> In general terms, it is to do away with sufferings of the sick, to lessen the
> violence of their diseases, and refuse to treat those who are overmas-
> tered by their diseases, realizing that in such cases medicine is power-
> less. . . . For if a man demand from an art a power over what does not
> belong to the art, or from nature a power over what does not belong to
> nature, his ignorance is more allied to madness than to lack of knowl-
> edge. (p. 234)

He concludes by saying that "unless we as physicians recognize
our limitations and the moral responsibility to administer our

services and technology in a compassionate and reasonable manner, we run the risk of being (as Hippocrates stated it) 'allied to madness'" (Wooley, 1991, p. 234).

The great Middle Ages physician Maimonides was invoked by Dr. Gene Stollerman in 1986, then the editor-in-chief of the *Journal of the American Geriatrics Society*, in an editorial in the journal titled "Lovable Decisions: Re-Humanizing Dying." He began by asking, "What has happened to the role of the physician as the steward of his patient's death?" (p. 172). He went on to quote Maimonides, who prayed, "Thou hast chosen me in thy grace, to watch over the life *and* death of thy creatures. I am about to fulfill my duties. Guide me in this immense work so that it may be of avail" (p. 172) (Stollerman, 1986). A recent review of Sir William Osler's involvement with death, as a part of his practice and study of medicine, appeared in the *Annals of Internal Medicine* (Hinohara, 1993). In it he is quoted as saying that patients will die in peace if they are looked after by "good physicians" who will act so that "when he can keep life no longer in, he makes a fair and easy passage of it to go out" (Osler, 1911, p. 740).

Other papers have been written to pursue the sources of physicians' preoccupation with life and aversion to death. Some suggest that certain personalities with a higher than normal fear of death enter the profession in efforts to overpower their fear (Feifel, 1965). Another explanation was given by Jean Benoliel (1974) in an article titled "Anticipatory Grief," in which she explored the professional losses associated with death, which include the loss of power and control over death; the need to confront possible errors in judgment that led to the death; the possible loss of respect from one's peers because a patient has died; the fact that dying situations threaten the controlled demeanor felt to be so important to the physician; the loss of a "significant patient," defined as someone in whom the practitioner has invested a good deal of time, energy, and clinical effort; and the loss of the social integration that attends a person's care (i.e., the temporary loss of purpose and collegiality the care of that patient gave).

The problem that arises when the physician has difficulty confronting death is the effect it has not only on the dying process for the patient, the staff, and the family but on the evaluative process that leads to that point at which further treatments appear futile and should not be continued or evidence exists that the person would not want medical treatment in his or her current state.

Nothing challenges the knowledge and wisdom of a physician more than trying to determine when treatment can no longer serve any useful purpose. Clearly, the path of least resistance is to err in favor of continued treatment. But although there is continuing disagreement over exactly what constitutes futility, there is general agreement that we should not subject patients to clearly futile treatments. And indeed, there is a growing societal mandate to limit such treatments in the name of cost containment. It therefore seems incumbent upon the profession to continue to pursue a common definition or at least guidelines in this area before someone else does it for us. Even where the task of making decisions to limit treatment is somewhat simplified by advance directives or surrogate decision makers, much care must be taken to adequately evaluate all evidence of patient wishes and continued capacity to participate in decision making, as well as the current medical condition and whether it warrants invoking treatment-limiting decisions. These tasks of establishing futility or patient wishes in the circumstance at hand require an objectivity that *cannot* exist if physicians have not reconciled their own feelings regarding death, not only for themselves but for their patients.

It has been written that physicians share "the same fear of death that other members of our society share" (Feldman, 1987, pp. 104–105). Medical training and practice have done little to address this fear since Dr. Kaspar's 1959 article. George Dickinson (1985) did a study from 1975 to 1985 on death education in U.S. medical schools. In this period, the number of medical school courses in death education increased only slightly. In 1975, there were 7 full-term courses in 113 medical schools. This rose to 16 out of 128 in 1980 but dropped to 14 out of 126 in 1985. Otherwise, occasional lectures and short courses were present in approximately 80% of the schools over the decade (Dickinson, 1985). Data from another study, however, suggests that these lectures occur mostly in the preclinical years of medical school, not during patient care rotations, when they would be more useful (Rappaport & Witzke, 1993). Data from the 1990–1991 *Association of American Medical Colleges Curriculum Directory* states that only 6 of 123 medical schools have a required course on death and dying. There are more mandatory geriatrics courses and an equal number of required computer courses in medical school, to put this in perspective. As an aside, there are 43 required courses in medical ethics (Association of American Medical Colleges, 1990–91). The education leading to ethical decision making is only half the battle. A major struggle continues in implementing the decision that a person should be allowed to die without further medical intervention. This is where personal feelings and doubts that death *can* be a best alternative really come into play, as the dying process is observed. It is not clear whether dealing with the dying process is included in these ethics courses, but it should be.

The literature suggests that physicians at all levels of training and practice are receptive to more training and guidance on death and dying and would indeed welcome it (Dickinson, 1988, Rappaport & Witzke, 1993). These efforts have to begin, however, from the starting point that (1) physicians are not more than human when it comes to feelings about death and dying and that (2) little has been provided in either the education or culture of medicine in the past few decades to address these feelings and reconcile them with good and compassionate medical care.

When physicians and other health care providers encounter discomfort with the dying process, Humphrey (1986) suggests a list of grief tasks. These include accepting the loss of ability to control death, finding satisfaction with patient-family comfort rather than cure, recognizing and adjusting to dynamics precipitated by loss, maintaining objectivity and therapeutic balance between patient and self, recognizing the eventual need of changing focus from dying patient to family members, adjusting to conflicting demands of others (patient, family, health team members, administration), and recognizing potential for his or her own grief and learning to seek appropriate help from others when needed. I would also suggest adding to the education process the lack of existing evidence that there is a professional mandate to provide medical treatments until death and that there are legal ramifications of providing unwanted treatments. In addition to education directed toward physicians and other health care providers, there should be made available a service or a professional in death and dying that can aid the physician and health care team in decisions to terminate treatment, as well as how best to facilitate the treatment termination.

Education must also be directed toward enhancing discussions about life and death between physicians and patients, with emphasis on the comfort that such knowledge can bring to the continuing care of a patient. For example, most physicians, when asked, appreciate the existence of advance directives in facilitating end-of-life decision making (Davidson, Hackler, Caradine, & McCord, 1989; Orentlicher, 1990). Yet one of the most commonly mentioned obstacles to their use is lack of physician-initiative in discussing them with patients (Finucane, Shumway, Powers, & D'Alessandri, 1988; Kohn & Menon, 1988; Lo et al., 1986). There are many reasons cited for this reluctance, but a major one is clearly the fact that the discussions involve death (La Puma, Orentlicher, & Moss, 1991; McIntyre, 1992).

Others have cited strategies to help physicians cope with death, including a very moving piece by a Dr. Lockhart McGuire (1990), who essentially wrote to describe how caring for dying patients and their families has enriched his professional life but also to share with others how he accomplished that care without experiencing mental exhaustion. In addition to technical confidence, listening to patients and the knowledge that gave him, and a humility about medical control of disease, he adds that physicians need some source of inner strength that identifies value in a life in terms other than how many years it has been lived or its physical or intellectual competence. He states that it does not have to come from organized religion, but it does have to be something important enough to make us willing to let go, both for ourselves and the dying patient, without feeling defeated and to make us feel that the value of our lives are not wholly extinguished by our deaths (McGuire, 1990). Osler, too, felt a similar sense of immortality important to his work with dying patients (Hinohara, 1993). How we encourage or facilitate such values in our caregivers is problematic but points to the need for some sort of spiritual guidance and support for staff involved in treatment termination.

What about the family? As alluded to, one of the major reasons for making the physician comfortable with the dying process, especially in situations in the nursing home where treatments are being terminated, is to provide the adequate support and guidance families need to help them make what they feel is the best decision for their family member and to ensure that the decision will be carried out in the most comfortable and humane manner possible. Families who are in a position to be surrogate decision makers can make decisions only as good as the information they receive from the health care team about medical conditions, prognoses, and the degree of comfort or discomfort attending various treatment options. As mentioned before, the physician plays a crucial role in the assessment of this information. For a family member who is committed to withdrawing or withholding therapy, the physician must be able to convey in an objective fashion what the process will most likely be like and what he or she plans to do to ensure patient comfort. He or she must in *some* situations employ interventions that address the family member's perceptions of pain or discomfort, even when these are not shared by the others involved in the patient's care. In our experience, even the family members who feel the *most* certain that treatment termination is consistent with their relative's wishes find the dying process more painful than they expected. They need the support of all of the staff, including the physician, in this process, sometimes for days to weeks following death. Medical tradition reflects this role of providing support during death, and physicians should not abandon it.

Another issue regarding family that sometimes arises in the nursing home is disagreement over the appropriateness of treatment termination between the real or biological family of a nursing home resident and the nursing home staff, who have also grown attached to the resident and become, in essence, a surrogate family. In many instances, staff members have seen themselves as having taken over the burden of care for the resident and do not understand family requests to limit treatments on the resident's behalf, especially when they perceive the resident to be comfortable (i.e., not suffering from whatever treatments are sustaining life). Families do not always recognize the relationships that develop between staff and nursing home residents and do not appreciate it when staff members raise concerns about the appropriateness of requests to limit treatment. We usually tell families that staff feelings will not guide our decision away from what appears to be the decision most consistent with the resident's wishes, but we do occasionally ask for time to deal with staff discomfort, so that staff members may move on with caring for the residents and their families, especially when treatments are being terminated.

A primary goal of educational efforts in ethics should be to illustrate to the staff that everyone's views of life and death are different and that to provide ongoing compassionate care they must accept these differences. The goal should not be to change staff views of life and death but to allow them to engage in behaviors that recognize and support this diversity. As David Thomasma (1987) puts it, respect for life does not always mean prolonging it. Physicians and philosophers have argued that the best way to respect life is to respect the values of those who possess that life. Again, as Thomasma (1987) states, "Nothing can be so cruel during one's dying than to lose one's values along with one's life" (p. 703).

## REFERENCES

Association of American Medical Colleges. (1990-91). *AAMC curriculum directory*. Washington, DC: Author.

Benoliel, J. Q. (1974). Anticipatory grief in physicians and nurses. In B. Schoenberg, A. C. Carr, A. H. Kutscher, D. Peretz, & I. K. Goldberg (Eds.), *Anticipatory grief*. New York: Columbia University Press.

Cohen-Mansfield, J., Rabinovich, B. A., Lipson, S., Fein, A., Gerber, B., Weisman, S. & Pawlson, L. G. (1991). The decision to execute a durable power of attorney for health care and preferences regarding the utilization of life-sustaining treatments in nursing home residents. *Archives of Internal Medicine, 151*, 289-294.

Davidson, K. W., Hackler, C., Caradine, D. R., & McCord, R. S. (1989). Physicians' attitudes on advance directives. *Journal of the American Medical Association, 262*, 2415-2419.

Dickinson, G. E. (1985). Changes in death education in U.S. medical schools during 1975-1985. *Journal of Medical Education, 60*(12), 942-943.

Dickinson, G. E. (1988). Death education for physicians. *Journal of Medical Education, 63*(5), 412.

Emanuel, L. L., Barry, M. J., Stoeckle, J. D., Ettelson, L. M., & Emanuel, E. J. (1991). Advance directives for medical care—a case for greater use. *New England Journal of Medicine, 324*(13), 889-895.

Feifel, H. 1965. The function of attitudes toward death. *Death and Dying: Attitudes of Patient and Doctor, 5*(11), 632-641.

Feldman, A. (1987). The dying patient. *Psychiatric Clinics of North America, 10*(1), 101-108.

Finucane, T. E., Shumway, J. M., Powers, R. L., & D'Alessandri, R. M. (1988). Planning with elderly outpatients for contingencies of severe illness. *Journal of General Internal Medicine, 3*, 322-325.

Hinohara, S. (1993). Sir William Osler's philosophy on death. *Annals of Internal Medicine, 118*(8), 638-642.

Humphrey, M. (1986). Effects of anticipatory grief for the patient, family member, and caregiver. In Rando, T. (Ed.) *Loss and anticipatory grief*. Lexington, MA: D.C. Heath.

Kaspar, A. M. (1959). The doctor and death. In Feifel, H. (Ed.), *The meaning of death* (pp. 259-270). New York: McGraw-Hill.

Kaye, J. M. (1988). The physician's role with the terminally ill patient. *Clinics in Geriatric Medicine, 4*(1), 13–27.

Kohn, M., & Menon, G. (1988). Life prolongation: Views of elderly outpatients and health care professionals. *Journal of the American Geriatrics Society, 36*, 840–844.

Kubler-Ross, E. (1969). *On death and dying.* New York: Macmillan.

La Puma, J., Orentlicher, D., & Moss, R. J. (1991). Advance directives on admission: Clinical implications and analysis of the Patient Self-Determination Act of 1990. *Journal of the American Medical Association, 266*(3), 402–405.

Lo, B., McLeod, G. A., & Saika, G. (1986). Patient attitudes to discussing life-sustaining treatment. *Archives of Internal Medicine, 146*, 1613–1615.

McGuire, L. B. (1990, Winter). Ourselves and patients who are dying. *The Pharos,* pp. 6–8.

McIntyre, K. M. (1992). Sheparding the patient's right to self-determination: The physician's dawning role. *Archives of Internal Medicine, 152*, 259–261.

Orentlicher, D. (1990). Advance medical directives. *Journal of the American Medical Society, 263*, 2365–2367.

Osler, W. (1911). Maeterlinck on death. *Spectator, 57*, 740.

Rappaport, W., & Witzke, D. (1993). Education about death and dying during the clinical years of medical school. *Surgery, 113*(2), 163–165.

Stollerman, G. H. (1986). Lovable decisions: Re-humanizing dying. *Journal of the American Geriatrics Society, 34*, 172–174.

Thomasma, D. C. (1987). Caveat philosophus: Technology's abuse-potential in the decision to terminate life. *Journal of the American Geriatrics Society, 35*, 703–704.

Wooley, M. W. (1991). Allied to madness [letter]. *Annals of Internal Medicine, 115*, 234.

## THE CASE OF MR. D

Mr. D is an 89-year-old man with heart disease and diabetes who has resided in your nursing home for several years. Some time ago, he suffered a stroke, which affected his ability to communicate. His only child, a daughter, is concerned that, should her father's condition worsen, he might receive more aggressive treatment than she believes he would prefer. You attempt to elicit from Mr. D what he would like to have done should he need additional treatment, but he is unable to tell you.

Although Mr. D never executed an advance directive, his daughter has produced strong evidence to indicate that Mr. D. would want her to make treatment decisions for him should he be unable to do so for himself. Further, you and your staff believe that the daughter has her father's best interests at heart. Accordingly, you agree to go along with Mr. D's daughter's wishes regarding treatment. Mr. D's daughter tells you and the primary health care team responsible for his care that she wants "no aggressive medical treatments" for her father and essentially wants him to receive only comfort care.

One weekend, when a covering physician unfamiliar with all of the specifics of the case is on duty, it is discovered that Mr. D has a dangerously high blood sugar level. The covering physician transfers Mr. D to the hospital on an emergency basis. When Mr. D's daughter becomes aware of this, she is very upset because she felt that hospitalization was more than comfort care. In addition, she wanted her father to remain in your nursing home among people he knows.

Upon his return to your facility, all involved in Mr. D's care agreed that comfort care should be their highest priority in his case. However, the physician on the primary care team is very reluctant not to treat Mr. D. She becomes concerned when Mr. D stops eating and she tells the daughter that tube feeding will keep her father more comfortable. However, the doctor is unable to control Mr. D's blood sugars after tube feeding is instituted.

The physician starts an IV and draws frequent blood sugar samples. However, Mr. D continues to go downhill and develops pneumonia. Because antibiotics will relieve many uncomfortable symptoms in addition to treating the pneumonia, Mr. D's daughter agrees to go along with their use. The pneumonia resolves, but Mr. D subsequently develops gangrene in his right leg. Mr. D's daughter is adamantly against amputation and asks that nothing more be done and that every attempt be made simply to keep her father comfortable with pain medication. Mr. D's primary care physician still feels strongly that she not only must continue to treat the pain but also must actively continue to treat Mr. D's other clinical problems. The rest of Mr. D's primary health care team would like to keep Mr. D as comfortable as possible, stop both the IV and blood drawing, and give Mr. D pain medication as needed. Mr. D's physician continues to disagree with the part of the care plan that the rest of the team wants to implement. When asked why, she tells you that by not continuing to treat all problems she is killing Mr. D.

## QUESTIONS FOR DISCUSSION

1. Why is it important to try to elicit an opinion from Mr. D regarding his treatment preferences?
2. What methods of communicating with Mr. D might be useful?
3. Absent advance directives, how can you determine who should make treatment decisions for Mr. D?
4. How can you determine that these decisions are in Mr. D's best interest?
5. Do you agree with Mr. D's physician? If not, what approach would you take with the patient and the doctor?

## ANSWERS

Eliciting information from exceedingly frail older persons who suffer from a variety of sensory and functional disabilities often is more easily said than done and frequently requires creative methods of communicating. For example, if oral questioning using the simplest possible terms yields no response from Mr. D, questions can be written down in large letters and shown to him. Every attempt must be made to elicit treatment preferences directly from Mr. D to assure his health care providers that they are indeed respecting his autonomy. This should be done in all cases in which the limitation of life-sustaining treatments is being considered, even in those cases where the patient's wishes had been previously delineated in a living will or where a health care agent had been named to make decisions.

Mr. D's was a case of double jeopardy. Not only was it impossible to ascertain his current treatment preferences directly from him, but he had never executed any type of advance directive. Therefore, it was necessary to determine not only what he would want as far as treatment is concerned but also who he would wish to make decisions for him.

Ascertaining who is the most appropriate treatment decision maker for a decisionally impaired older person is easier in some cases than in others. In the case of Mr. D, there was no spouse and only one child. When other, more distant relatives and friends were questioned, their unanimous agreement that Mr. D would have wanted his daughter to be his decision maker made things relatively easy. However, the literature (Molloy, Clarnette, Braun, Eisemann, & Schneiderman, 1991) and anecdotal reports suggest that things are not always so simple, particularly when there are several potential decision makers who cannot come to a unanimous agreement. Here, it is sometimes useful to refer these individuals to an ethics committee or utilize some other mechanism to resolve their dispute.

Clearly, making life-sustaining treatment decisions for those who have not left evidence of their wishes is fraught with difficulties. When faced with decisions for which there is no prior information about patient wishes, one must rely on a "best interest" standard (Beauchamp & Childress, 1989; Emanuel, 1987). This relies not only on what the majority of people in a similar situation would want but is also based on the evaluation of the relative benefits and burdens of the proposed treatment(s). Even in these situations, patient values obviously come into play, and the family or others who know the patient well are probably in the best position to make these determinations. If, however, the choices made by the family seem unreasonable or unjustified, given the relative risks of a treatment compared to the potential benefits, then the health care team has an obligation to challenge the family. In this case, Mr. D is suffering from a progressive downhill course despite reasonably aggressive therapy. Requesting that medical interventions beyond comfort care be discontinued in a case such as this does not appear to transcend the boundaries of a reasonable course of action. Therefore, there appears to be little reason to challenge the daughter's request.

Another problem that arises in cases involving treatment termination centers on the feelings of the health care providers involved in the case, most notably members of the medical and nursing professions. These individuals and their paraprofessional counterparts, nursing aides or nursing assistants, often regard the termination of life-sustaining treatment as antithetical to their training. Accordingly, they may need a great deal of support and education when a patient opts to forgo life-sustaining treatment.

Mr. D's physician is a case in point. She needs counseling and support regarding her role as a caregiver, with emphasis on the fact that being able to recognize when further treatment may be futile, as well as inconsistent with the patient's wishes, is as much a part of her responsibilities as providing aggressive medical care.

If the physician cannot reconcile her personal beliefs regarding her professional obligations, she should be offered the opportunity to transfer care of the resident to another doctor, who is willing to abide by the resident's and family's wishes. The primary goal should be, however, to help Mr. D's physician recognize that not all people want the same level of treatment at the end of their lives and that such variability is acceptable, both ethically and legally. Hopefully, such understanding will enable this physician to provide good care to all of her patients, regardless of their specific treatment preferences.

## REFERENCES

Beauchamp, T. L., & Childress, J. F. (1989). *Principles of biomedical ethics* (3rd. ed.). New York: Oxford University Press.

Emanuel, E. J. (1987, October–November). A communal vision of care for incompetent patients. *Hastings Center Report*, pp. 15–20.

Molloy, D. W., Clarnette, R. M., Braun, E. A., Eisemann, M. R., & Schneiderman, B. (1991). Decision making in the incompetent elderly: "The Daughter from California Syndrome." *Journal of the American Geriatrics Society, 39*, 396–399.

# 5

# Home Versus Nursing Home: Getting Beyond the Differences

*Bart J. Collopy*

For the elderly and their families facing decisions about long-term care, the choice that shapes almost all others is the choice between nursing home care and care at home. The choice is generally framed as a polarity, a stark opposition: home *versus* nursing home. This brisk either/or summons up, on one side, our moral passion for autonomy and privacy and independence; on the other side, our wariness about institutional control, our fears of dependency and collective living. The polarity is further reenforced by the present health care system—short on fiscal resources, staggered by the prospect of an aging population, and anxious to establish clear (one might say "forbidding") boundaries between expensive nursing home care and less-costly community-based care.

The home versus nursing home schema suggests, then, a sharp divide between care at home and care in an institution. The cultural view of nursing homes as grim keeps of the elderly seems unshakable, even though much of it is based on past history rather than current reality, on worst-case examples rather than more typical ones (Collopy, Boyle, & Jennings, 1991; Gubrium, 1975; Vladeck, 1980).

On the other hand, even if these misperceptions are corrected, nursing home care remains a moral thicket. And passage through this thicket is no easy walk. Care providers know that moral tangles are constant and common stuff in institutional long-term care. Residents confront the loss of familiar settings and routines and social contacts; they hope to preserve independence and privacy, to reassemble some version of the daily freedoms they knew when living in their own homes.

Within the home versus nursing home polarity, these are the kinds of issues that influence us away from nursing home care, that make care at home seem like such an absolute better choice. But the concerns about life in the nursing home, whether real or imagined, are hardly the best reasons for esteeming home care. In fact, valuation of this sort is liable to overlook the *institutional* affinities between these two forms of care. Despite its community setting, home care abounds with institutional structures, with its own thick web of regulations and restrictions, eligibility rules and reimbursement processes, provider and vendor subsystems, hierarchies of assessment, supervision, and review.

Whereas nursing homes are often depicted as the culprit places in long-term care precisely because of their institutional character, the institutionalized aspects of home care seem to escape public attention. Perhaps our romanticized notions of "home" and "family" are responsible for this, creating a rosy myopia about home care that only heightens our bleak cultural images of nursing homes. This double blurring serves community-based care no better than institutional care. Home care has allowed a significant number of people to remain at home with appropriate and compassionate care. However, the blunt, unromanticized fact is that in a system with tightly limited resources many of the elderly may be kept out of nursing homes but with a level of community care that does not allow them to flourish in any real sense (Cohen, 1988; Kane, 1989; Hennessy, 1989).

Staying at home might come, then, at the price of having fewer resources and supports than would be available in a nursing facility. In such straits, "independence" translates into an elderly person alone and isolated, struggling to manage with far from optimal medical and nursing and personal assistance. As frailty progresses, "home" may tighten into a narrow box of a world. Family caregivers may find themselves overwhelmed by burdens they never anticipated. The moral basis and limits of family obligations may grow unclear, the caregiving relationship wither into a dread linkage of guilt (Callahan, 1987).

It seems, then, that any cataloging of hard questions about institutional care should be counterbalanced by questions about home care. For example, will the hospital discharge process force me into a home care plan that leaves me insecure and unsafe? Will home care put too many burdens on my family? What will this do to cherished relationships, to already frayed ones? Will home care providers be reluctant to take me as a client if I want to go on living in my fourth-floor walk-up in a deteriorating neighborhood or if I refuse to have my apartment cleaned or my three dogs walked more regularly? What will happen if my care providers think my home is cluttered and unsafe and unsanitary, while I find in its mess the map of my life? And if my family cares for me poorly, treats me shabbily, even abusively, will care providers respect my refusal to report this, to do *anything* about it? Will they accept my explanation that this is my family even though we battle, sometimes harshly?

## COMMON GROUND, RATHER THAN DEEP DIVIDE

These questions suggest that the divide between home care and institutional care might not be so vast, that both forms of care face puzzles about autonomy and beneficence, safety and independence, conflict and lack of congruence between the values of the elderly and their caregivers (Zuckerman, Dubler, & Collopy, 1990; Haddad & Kapp, 1991; Kane & Caplan, 1992). Long-term care ethics should, then, draw out the common ground, the shared ethical struggles that link institutional and home care. It is commonplace to argue that long-term care is best served through an integrated continuum of services rather than a fragmented, atomistic, scatter of resources. So too, the *ethics* of long-term care is best served through a continuum of moral concerns, a sense of the common moral ground shared by institutional and community-based forms of care.

To suggest what this common ground might look like, I will briefly examine seven areas where the elderly and their families face problems that deserve common ethical reflection from both nursing homes and home care agencies.

## Becoming a Client or Resident

Entry into long-term care can mean that the elderly and their families must confront complex and confusing information, tight decision-making deadlines, and a very limited, perhaps fear-laden, view of the road ahead. Care providers may press the decision-making process forward to meet their own obligations and deadlines. And they may—from beneficence or paternalism or sheer pragmatics—urge a particular long-term care option, perhaps present it more as a given than an option. Along with these pressures, families may find themselves struggling with internal tensions and disagreements, with the puzzles of role changes and reversals.

The end result can be a placement or admissions process dominated on one side by family members or other "responsible parties" and on the other side by discharge planners, case managers, and staff members responsible for assessment and admissions. This leaves home care agencies and nursing homes with some common ethical questions. How can the voice of the elderly person be preserved—directly or by really effective surrogacy—in the midst of the placement process? How can care providers manage the pressures of the health care system—and the subsystems of their own facilities and agencies—so that the values, goals, and expectations of the elderly client or resident effectively shape the placement process?

## Preserving the Freedoms of Daily Life

For the elderly in nursing homes or home care the basic quality of care is liable to be defined in the caregiving related to the activities of daily life (ADL) or instrumental activities of daily life (IADL). These activities (e.g., eating, moving about, bathing, dressing, toileting, shopping, housekeeping, managing money) do not produce the immediate moral drama of decisions about end-of-life tube feeding or assisted suicide. But in long-term care it is the seemingly mundane that often tells the tale of human autonomy and dignity.

It is crucial, then, that nursing homes and home care agencies look beyond the ethics of Do Not Resuscitate (DNR) orders and tube feeding and advance directives to those ADL and IADL issues that fill the months and years before a patient's final hours. This wider ethical focus will not come easily in a health care system that instinctively medicalizes care, reducing the protean realities of aging to categories of disease and illness (Estes & Binney, 1989). The long-term care sector faces an uphill task in developing an ethics agenda that gives high priority to daily life issues, that assertively reflects the *psychosocial* dimensions of care.

## Taking Risks

Some of the hardest conflicts in long-term care arise when elderly individuals make decisions or behave in ways that family members, care providers, regulators, or even the surrounding community find unsafe or disruptive (Hennessey, 1989; Kane & Caplan, 1992). In a health care system that has traditionally made safety a hierarch among values, how can providers recognize risk taking as a normal element in adult life, an inalienable part of being autonomous, even when one is elderly and frail? What boundaries —or better, what *tolerances*—should long-term care develop for the "behavioral outliers," for individuals who are sharply singular or eccentric, who persistently breach social decorum and convention? How should providers balance the right of elderly individuals to take risks with their own obligations to protect these individuals from harm—and from harming others? How should they weigh an individual's autonomy against the common good of the institutional or local community?

In the past, the routine use of physical and chemical restraints suggested that "problematic" behavior on the part of the frail elderly should be automatically curbed. Within the past 5 years a strong ethical, regulatory, and "best practice" consensus has rejected this notion. From an ethical perspective, routine use of restraints means routine restriction of personal autonomy and dignity (Collopy, 1992). Restraints can, moreover, exacerbate disruptive behavior and leave behind a trail of physical and psychological damage (Evans & Strumpf, 1989). In professional terms, the routine use of restraints straitjackets providers, tying them to a desperately small repertoire of responses to a wide range of harmful and disruptive behavior.

Recent efforts to reduce the use of restraints have produced a wide range of alternatives, indicating that ethical challenges to accepted patterns of care can widen the knowledge base of the field and advance standards of practice. The ethical challenge here is, of course, not directed merely at restraints but at the wider issues of behavior management in long-term care. This larger issue presents providers with the task of developing models of practice that value safety, medical priorities, and communal quality of life but do not absolutize any of these values, do not impose on care providers some unreal norm of risk-free and disturbance-free care.

## Facing Loss of Mental Capacity

An assessment of cognitive incapacity in an elderly client or resident means a corresponding loss of autonomy. But how should care providers respond when there is a lingering sense of autonomy in residents or clients with mental incapacity? How should providers care for individuals who suffer serious cognitive loss but *still* have preferences and choices, still feel they must make decisions, take care of things, worry about responsibilities, perform chores, go places, do what they have always done?

Here the basic philosophical and psychological issue is the relationship between outer behavior and the inner dynamics of the self experiencing cognitive loss (Foley, 1992). When this inner self is not immediately or clearly present, what kind of practical impact should it have on the hectic flow of daily care routines? Even when it is quite impenetrable, should the inner self of the incapacitated person speak some lingering claim on care providers, requiring at least that they proceed with deep caution and reluctance whenever they step in and override an individual's choice or behavior?

These questions reveal the critical *ethical* dimensions of assessments of mental capacity. Because individuals' moral agency is curtailed when they are judged incapacitated or incompetent, the reliability of such assessments requires careful and constant scrutiny. Assessments can be skewed by cultural and professional expectations about the prevalence of dementia among the frail elderly. Or the inability of frail elderly to execute choices can be taken as a sign of incapacity to *make* choices. Or noncompliance, refusal of treatment, idiosyncratic behavior can be seen as "evidence" of mental incapacity. Even diagnostic language can produce blur rather than precision. Functioning as blanket categories, "dementia" or "Alzheimer's" may simply cover over the wide differences in elderly individuals with the same diagnosis.

Assessments of capacity play an equally central role in home care and institutional care and suggest a common effort to develop more rigorous and differentiated sorts of assessments. This would mean moving beyond mental status tests and other initial screenings to more thorough testing for reversible causes of confusion, more careful efforts to track fluctuating mental capacity, to define capacity in terms of specific decisions or areas of behavior. For this to be effective, agencies and facilities would have to develop policies that set a consistent organizational standard for assessing capacity and for regularly reviewing such assessments.

## Making Medical Treatment Decisions

Long-term care now faces complex ethical questions about medical treatment, especially in the area of terminal care. These questions are extensively and expertly discussed by other articles in this collection, and I will therefore not comment on them—except for a reminder, now at least mildly ideological, from "Preserving the Freedoms of Daily Life," above.

The complexities of medical treatment decisions understandably dominate clinical ethics in acute care. But long-term care should be wary of replicating this. By definition, long-term *care* reaches far beyond *medical treatment*. The daily ethical conflicts in chronic care are not limited to medical treatment, certainly not to terminal care. Long-term care ethics ought, then, to develop its own indigenous agenda, define and explore its own spectrum of issues. While dealing with the important issues of medical treatment and terminal care, it should give high priority to exploring issues that relate to daily life care, the special needs of the frail elderly and their families, and the diverse moral imperatives that come with a psychosocial model of care.

## Dealing with Organizational Structures

Becoming a home care client or nursing home resident means stepping into a world of powerful organizational patterns and structures—at a point in life when one may feel particularly unarmed and vulnerable. Awareness of this power imbalance is a crucial gauge of the moral sensibilities of any facility or agency.

In short, the ethics of care require reflection on and control of institutional clout.

There is, of course, an irony here. The power of a caregiving organization is most effectively scrutinized and checked by the organization itself. Individual staff members can (and should) work against what is impersonal and inflexible in the structures of care, but their success in this will be localized and transient, a kind of guerilla ethic, if the organization itself remains unconcerned and unchanged. Although the moral sensibilities and commitments of staff members are absolutely essential to the ethics of care, *corporate* moral agency is not simply the sum of these individual sensibilities. On the contrary, if there is little formal, structural attention to ethical issues, staff members are liable to feel that their moral quandaries and struggles have low priority, that "the organization" is concerned uppermost with the logistics, legalities, and fiscal ledgers of care.

Both the workings of the health care system and the intrinsic ambiguities of caring for dependent elderly make for obvious tension between the managerial and moral concerns of care-providing organizations. This tension can be of a creative sort, but this requires tangible expenditures of time and energy—efforts to make and monitor policies around ethical issues, ongoing educational programs and in-service training, institutional mechanisms to help staff with morally difficult cases, and such things as ethics rounds, ethics-consulting teams, and institutional ethics committees (Brown, Miles, & Aroskar, 1987; Libow et al., 1992; Olson et al., 1993; Thompson & Thompson, 1990; Zweibel & Cassel, 1988).

Organizational response to ethical issues requires particular attention to the paraprofessional staff. In both nursing homes and home care programs, these staff members provide the bulk of daily hands-on care. From a productivity standpoint, their work can be measured in a catalog of "bed and body" tasks (Lidz & Arnold, 1990). But from an ethical standpoint this is painfully narrow, even obtuse. Daily personal care shapes the ethical environment of a facility or agency. For the elderly themselves this care is liable to carry intensely personal relational meaning. On both sides of these relationships, problems can develop around issues of choice and control, dignity and competency, modes of authority and accommodation. Yet, in dealing with these conflicts, paraprofessional staff members, especially in home care, can feel isolated, left with little support and guidance, short of warnings about regulatory and liability risks.

A critical measure of an organization's commitment to the ethics of care is, then, its willingness to listen and respond to the moral difficulties that staff members face. In organizational terms, *response* means resources: in-service training, support and mediation from supervisors, opportunities for peer discussion and problem solving, and inclusion in care planning and in other aspects of organizational life, which would affirm all staff members' crucial contribution to the quality of care.

## Living in a World of Regulations

The regulatory system exerts strong control over long-term care, setting eligibility and reimbursement standards, monitoring everything from medical treatment and personal care to safety, cleanliness, and other physical aspects of the care setting. The resulting standardization reduces the freedom of the elderly to personalize their care, to take risks, choose providers, and shape schedules and other caregiving arrangements to their own preferences. If they seek to cut their own autonomous paths across the system, the elderly may find that care providers are reluctant to assist them, even when the providers morally agree with their challenge to the letter of the law. In short, the regulation of nursing homes and home care programs inevitably means the regulation of elderly residents and clients.

In the way it shapes the moral environment of care, regulation is a crucial concern for both providers and the elderly they care for. Inevitably, regulation defines quality of care in the "measurables" that are the stuff of on-site inspections and record reviews. This checklist approach provides systematic checks against substandard care. It allows regulators to monitor changing standards of practice, to press providers whose care may be borderline, to build a detailed case against those whose care is inadequate.

But this mode of regulation fixates on infractions, creating an environment in which regulators are accusatory, providers anxious and self-defensive. Rather than lifting ethical sensibilities, regulation by inspection tends to set legal and minimalistic norms. Thus, providers describe regulation as an outside force imposing unrealistic, costly bureaucratic burdens that stifle professional initiative and standardize patient care. It might be suggested that this response is to be expected from providers—the supervised bristling at their overseers. But if it is expected, inevitable, "natural," this sense of alienation only underscores how deeply systemic the problem is. At its heart, by its very *structure*, the present system is adversarial. It favors punitive force over persuasion, control over consensus, mandating outcomes over seeding ethical motivations.

Nursing homes and home care agencies face a common hazard here. An adversarial regulatory system instinctively views providers as members of an industry that has to be tightly regulated because it is potentially *harmful* to its vulnerable elderly consumers. Thus, the regulatory system must define the ethics of care as *its* special preserve, and it must, accordingly, micromanage providers into ethically correct practice. The regulator looking over the shoulder of the care provider becomes the real guarantor of ethical care. In the end, the moral relationship between patients and care providers is marginalized, ethics is reduced to "following the regs," and the vulnerable elderly are left to the letter of the law. These morally corrosive, even if unintended, outcomes provide a powerful incentive for exploring the *ethical* ramifications of regulation. Analysis must focus on the moral ironies of the present regulatory system. Legislating and patrolling moral boundaries is an ambiguous undertaking when the goal is to assure high levels of *caregiving*.

In their concern to preserve richer notions of their own moral agency, institutional and home care providers face a common and large task: pressing the discussion of government regulation (and the discussion *with* government regulators) to the level of its *moral* premises and implications. Essential to this discussion is the need for a clear statement of providers' own moral concerns, their stake in advancing the issues now shaping the ethics agenda in long-term care.

## CONCLUSION: LONG-TERM CARE AND CULTURAL PERCEPTIONS OF ADVANCED AGE

In the world of bioethics, long-term care has lived something of a marginal existence, cutting its ethics from the cloth of acute care, largely from issues that cluster around autonomy (e.g., patient self-determination, medical decision making, informed consent, advance directives). This derivative position reflects, I suspect, a measure of intellectual disinterest, a presumption that long-term care does not offer enough precipice—medical or moral—for a challenging climb.

But there may be other factors operating here. It may not be a lack of moral or intellectual precipice that leaves long-term care ethics unexplored so much as an unwillingness to approach the precipices that are there. Long-term care deals daily and frontally with human frailty, with realities that our culture finds deeply discomforting. In short, nursing homes and home agencies challenge the cultural mind-set, our "activist" but repressive images of aging, our efforts to manage—and perhaps mask—our mortality.

From this perspective, long-term care does face a precipice but one we have little zest (or tools) to scale. "Frailty" seems, for example, such an imprecise category, etiologically loose, medically vague, and useless. Yet in its imprecision it looms large and complex, taking to itself all of the illnesses, disabilities, and impairments—physical, psychological, and social—that can unravel later life. It is a sheer cliff to theory and practice precisely because it evokes a moral condition as well as a physical one, a complex fate more akin to mortality or mutability than disease, closer to poverty than to prostate cancer, to finitude than to renal failure.

Showing *these* family resemblances, frailty raises large questions about selfhood and moral identity, about the endgames as well as the benefits of autonomy, the companioning tasks of caregiving, the spiritual ends of medicine and the other caring professions. Most of all, it raises questions about the meaning of advanced age. It reminds us that if long life is a gift to be happily and resolutely grasped, it often comes with the barb of diminishment and suffering. As a response to this paradox of the human condition, long-term care presses us to examine the darker aspect of aging, to challenge the presumption that longevity is pure boon. It also challenges those strains of biomedical ethics that find sufficient moral guide in the freedom of individuals to construe their own meaning and values for old age (as for any other stage of life). Such a view is strong in pressing procedural protections for individual choice, but it offers little substantive analysis of how, as a *community*, we construe the meaning of advanced age (Binstock & Post, 1991; Callahan, 1987; Homer & Holstein, 1990).

Bioethics has been quite tight-lipped about these larger issues, the need to explore the moral meaning of frailty and advanced age. Even gerontology has operated with great unprobed assumptions in this area. Advocacy for the elderly is the backbone of many of these assumptions, but advocacy is often too unsubtle and unsupple a concept to meet the complexities of aging and long-term care. Thus, activist images of aging may correct past stereotypes of elderly incapacity, but they also back away from the far side of aging, settling down in the territory of the young-old, where retirement and leisure rather than frailty and health care are the watchwords.

In the long run, then, the home versus nursing home polarity gives way to larger questions about the meaning of advanced age and caregiving, questions that provide the context for any particular decision we face about care setting, about the varying opportunities for autonomy that we might find in an institution or in the community. These larger questions caution us about focusing on the differences between nursing homes and home care agencies. They suggest that we look just as concertedly at basic definitions of frailty and caregiving, at the presumptions that provide the conceptual footing of long-term care. Here we find a vast tract of common ground. Long-term care ethics will best be served by institutional and community providers exploring this common ground together.

## REFERENCES

Binstock, R. H., & Post, S. G. (1991). *Too old for health care?* Baltimore: Johns Hopkins University Press.

Brown, B. A., Miles, S. H., & Aroskar, M. A. (1987). The prevalence and design of ethics committees in nursing homes. *Journal of the American Geriatrics Society, 35,* 1028–1033.

Callahan, D. (1987). *Setting limits: Medical goals in an aging society.* New York: Simon and Schuster.

Cohen, E. S. (1988). The elderly mystique: Constraints on the autonomy of the elderly with disabilities. *Gerontologist, 28*(Suppl.), 24–51.

Collopy, B. (1992). *The use of restraints in long-term care: The ethical issues.* Washington, DC: American Association of Homes for the Aging.

Collopy, B., Boyle, P., & Jennings, B. (1991). New directions in nursing home ethics. *Hastings Center Report, 21*(2, Suppl.), 1–16.

Estes, C. L., & Binney, E. A. (1989). The biomedicalization of aging: Dangers and dilemmas. *Gerontologist, 29,* 587–596.

Evans, L. K., & Strumpf, N. E. (1989). Tying down the elderly: A review of the literature on physical restraint. *Journal of the American Geriatric Society, 37,* 65–74.

Foley, J. M. (1992). The experience of being demented. In R. H. Binstock, S. G. Post, & P. J. Whitehouse (Eds.), *Dementia and aging: Ethics, values, and policy choices.* Baltimore: Johns Hopkins University Press.

Gubrium, J. F. (1975). *Living and dying at Murray Manor.* New York: St. Martin's Press.

Haddad, A. M., & Kapp, M. B. (1991). *Ethical and legal issues in home health care: Case studies and analyses.* Norwalk, CT: Appleton and Lange.

Hennessy, C. H. (1989). Autonomy and risk: The role of client wishes in community-based long-term care. *Gerontologist, 29,* 633–639.

Homer, P., & Holstein, M. (1990). *A good old age?* New York: Simon and Schuster.

Kane, N. M. (1989). The home care crisis of the nineties. *Gerontologist, 29,* 24–31.

Kane, R. A. & Caplan, A. L. (Eds.). (1992). *Ethical conflicts in the management of home care: The case manager's dilemma.* New York: Springer Publishing Co.

Libow, L. S., Olson, E., Neufeld, R. R., Martico-Greenfield, T., Meyers, H., Gordon, N., & Barnett, P. (1992). Ethics rounds at the nursing home: An alternative to an ethics committee. *Journal of the American Geriatrics Society, 40*(1), 94–97.

Lidz, C. W., & Arnold, R. M. (1990). Institutional constraints on autonomy. *Generations, 14,* 65–68.

Olson, E., Chichin, E. R., Libow, L. S., Martico-Greenfield, T., Neufeld, R. R., & Mulvihill, M. (1993). A center on ethics in long-term care. *Gerontologist, 33,* 269–274.

Thompson, M. A., & Thompson, J. M. (1990). Ethics committees in nursing homes: A qualitative research study. *Hospital Ethics Committee Forum, 2,* 315–327.

Vladeck, B. (1980). *Unloving care: The nursing home tragedy.* New York: Basic Books.

Zuckerman, C., Dubler, N. N., & Collopy, B. (Eds.). (1990). *Home health care options.* New York: Plenum Press.

Zweibel, N. R., & Cassel, C. K. (1988). Ethics committees in nursing homes: Applying the hospital experience. *Hastings Center Report, 18*(4), 23–25.

## THE CASE OF MS. E

Ms. E was admitted to your nursing home with a diagnosis of dementia and a long history of heart disease. It is obvious that her cognitive ability is markedly limited. Although cheerful, her verbal responses are inappropriate. In addition, she is unable to walk and spends most of her time out of bed in a wheelchair.

Ms. E had been admitted to your facility from the hospital. Prior to her admission to the hospital, her condition had been slowly deteriorating at home. For several months, her husband had cared for her with the assistance of a round-the-clock home attendant.

On admission to your nursing home, Ms. E's husband presents you with a health care proxy (in which he is named as agent) and a living will that outlines her requests for no life-sustaining treatments, including antibiotics, feeding tubes, and resuscitation. He tells you that, because he is named as agent and it is obvious that his wife is unable to make decisions, he is aware that his role as agent is now in effect. He also tells you that he does not want his wife to have any treatment or any diagnostic tests, including the basic laboratory tests that are routinely done on admission to your home. He feels her quality of life has fallen below an acceptable threshold, and besides, the doctors in the hospital gave her little hope of surviving more than a few weeks or months.

With time and much encouragement, Ms. E's husband agrees to the minimum admission testing but is very reluctant for her to receive any treatment whatsoever, even requesting that all cardiac medications be stopped. You deny this request, but agree to other limitations, such as "do not hospitalize." After a few months in your facility, however, Ms. E's physical condition improves without aggressive care to the extent that she is able to walk. In addition, her mental condition also shows some improvement. Although she is able to verbalize that she still enjoys life and does not object to medical treatment, you do not feel that she has the capacity to take charge of her care. At this time, Mr. E informs you that he is taking his wife home with 24-hour home care.

## QUESTIONS FOR DISCUSSION

1. Does Mr. E have the right to refuse routine admission tests for his wife?

2. How comfortable are you with Mr. E's decision to take his wife home?
3. Are you concerned about Ms. E's safety once she leaves your facility? If so, are you legally or ethically obliged to try to prevent her from leaving?


## ANSWERS

When Mr. E assumed the role of his wife's health care agent, he was given the same power to make health care decisions regarding treatment for his wife that she would have had if she had been decisionally capable. However, in determining exactly which decisions can or cannot be made, other factors must also be taken into consideration. For example, it may be acceptable for Mr. E to refuse to allow you to perform certain admission screening tests. However, if not performing those procedures has public health implications (e.g., routine admission tests for tuberculosis), those implications take precedence over Mr. E's wishes. Similarly, if you can ascertain that Mr. E is not acting in good faith by refusing certain tests or permitting certain treatments, his rights as a health care agent can be overruled. An assessment in this area would involve in part an evaluation of the relative risks and benefits of the therapies as well as their efficacy in prolonging life versus providing comfort. Although an agent may resist the life-sustaining aspect of cardiac medications, their administration results in little burden to the resident as long as they are carefully monitored. Further, their administration provides great benefit in terms of avoiding cardiac symptoms such as shortness of breath or chest pain. A similar argument could be made for antibiotics for a urinary tract infection that could be extremely painful but not immediately life-threatening. Refusal of treatment in these situations may well lead one to question Mr. E's intentions.

Although Mr. E has the legal right to take his wife home, his behavior while Ms. E was a resident in your facility may make you somewhat uneasy about her welfare after discharge. Here again you must be certain to at least some degree that her husband is acting in her best interest in taking her home. You, then, have a moral, if not a legal, responsibility to come to this determination. An approach might be to contact other available family members and the witnesses to Ms. E's proxy designation and living will to judge the seriousness of Ms. E's wishes, not only for limiting care but for entrusting her husband with decision making. If it clearly appears to be her wish to limit treatment in her current situation and to empower her husband to determine her best interests, despite your discomfort you most likely would have no grounds on which to challenge the discharge.

# 6

# Comfort Care in End-Stage Dementia: What to Do After Deciding to Do No More

*Ann C. Hurley,*
*Margaret A. Mahoney, and*
*Ladislav Volicer*

Currently, there is no known cure or way to prevent dementia of the Alzheimer type (DAT). In the later stages of the disease, inpatient care is nearly inevitable (Fabiszewski, Riley, Berkley, Karner, & Shea, 1988; U.S. Congress, 1990) and is often required for the last 3 years of life (Volicer et al., 1987). However, even inpatient care is limited in that it can offer only symptomatic treatment and the provision of a comfortable and safe environment (Maas, 1988) and does not affect the progressive and incurable nature of DAT.

The treatment of disease symptoms in the advanced stage poses ethical and clinical dilemmas (Volicer, 1986; Volicer & Fabiszewski, 1988; Volicer, Rheaume, Brown, Fabiszweski, & Brady, 1986). These dilemmas concern the use of aggressive medical interventions that may or may not extend a patient's life, often cause patient discomfort, increase the risk of precipitating iatrogenic complications, and drive up health care costs.

When providing optimal care to patients suffering with late-stage DAT, the decision faced by the family and treatment team should not be whether or not to stop treatment. This chapter

takes the position that the decision should be how much the paradigm should be changed from *high-tech* to *high-touch* care. Changing the paradigm means that the desired outcome is not maintaining life at all cost but is the process of maintaining patients'
comfort. In the high-touch paradigm, patients' surrogates, supported by the interdisciplinary health care team, make decisions
that direct the care of patients with DAT. Empowering patients
through their surrogates maintains the ethical principle of autonomy, integrates the values of the patient/family into the care
plan, preserves the dignity of the patient, and prevents loss of
control over the dying process.

Volicer (1986) suggested that a hospice philosophy, which re-
jects termination of suffering by suicide but provides palliative
care with a goal of maximal comfort and not maximal survival of
the patient, be applied to the care of end-stage DAT patients. In
summarizing the ethical perspective for providing palliative versus aggressive care for patients with advanced DAT, Volicer (1)
cited a statement adopted by the house of delegates of the American Medical Association on December 4, 1993, that permits ces-
sation of employment of extraordinary means to prolong life if
the patient or family agrees; (2) noted that it was generally accepted that a patient has a right to refuse treatment that is not
curative or that results in too great a burden; (3) stated that there
is no ethical reason why an individual has to be exposed to extraordinary medical interventions, resulting in greater suffering
just because he is demented; and (4) concluded that it should be
possible to limit medical interventions to provide comfort without striving for maximal survival in end-stage DAT patients, as it
is for terminal cancer patients.

This ethical stance has been made operational at the three
inpatient Dementia Special Care Units (DSCUs) managed by the
Geriatric Research Education and Clinical Center of the Edith
Nourse Rogers Memorial Veterans Hospital, Bedford, Massachusetts. A hospice philosophy of care, in which the patient's family
or legal guardian makes an advance decision regarding the extent of medical treatment to be provided or withheld (Volicer et
al., 1986), has been in place for almost a decade. Patients are
assigned to a level of medical intervention when the family
member(s) meets with the interdisciplinary team (family conference). This interdisciplinary team consists of the nursing unit
administrator and/or other nurses from the patient's unit, social
worker, nurse practitioner, chaplain, and attending physician. The

family conference is usually scheduled 6–8 weeks after admission to long-term care to give the family time to develop a trusting relationship with staff and for the clinical team to get to know the patient.

Prior to the conference, the nursing staff meets with the attending physician and develops a consensus regarding what the staff members consider the optimal level of care that should be recommended to the family. This consensus is used as a guideline for initiating the discussion with the family.

At the family conference, patients' surrogates are asked about any previous wishes the patient might have expressed regarding survival in a mentally and physically debilitated state or with the help of machines. The nursing staff recommendation of an optimal level of care is presented in terms of decisions regarding resuscitation, intensive support of failing physiologic function, fever management and the use of antibiotics, and artificial versus natural feeding. Families are assured that keeping patients comfortable, regardless of the level of medical intervention selected, is the primary goal of the DSCUs. That means, when a decision is made to forgo life-prolonging medical interventions, families are selecting intensive care nursing rather than high-tech medical care. Decisions reached are indicated on a form that is then signed by the patient's surrogate and all staff members who were present at the conference.

This is Advance Proxy Planning, which designates the scope of medical care to be carried out. The signed form states that family members may change their treatment decisions at any time. The form is placed in the patient's medical record, and the care limitations are specified on the physician's order sheet. The order is reviewed and renewed monthly. The family conference is repeated if the patient's condition changes substantially and/or at the request of the family. If the patient is placed on the seriously ill list, families are contacted and at that time have an opportunity to affirm or change any previous decisions. There are five levels of care.

*Level 1.* The patient receives aggressive diagnostic workups as indicated and treatment of coexisting medical conditions and is transferred to an acute care unit if necessary. In the event of cardiopulmonary arrest, resuscitation is attempted. Tube feeding is used if normal food intake is not possible.

*Level 2.* The patient receives complete medical care as defined, and here again, tube feeding is used if normal food intake is not possible. However, resuscitation is not attempted in the event of a cardiac or respiratory arrest. This requires a Do Not Resuscitate (DNR) order.

*Level 3.* The patient has a DNR order and is not transferred to an acute care unit for medical management of intercurrent life-threatening illnesses. This eliminates the use of intravenous treatments, respirators, cardiovascular support, and the like, which are available only in an acute-care medical setting. Transfers are made if required to maintain comfort (e.g., to set a broken hip), and tube feeding is used if normal food intake is not possible.

*Level 4.* The patient has a DNR order and is not transferred to an acute care unit. In addition, if the patient develops a fever, there is no diagnostic workup or antibiotic treatment for life-threatening infections (pneumonia, urinary tract infection). Liberal antipyretics and analgesics are used to ensure patient comfort. Oral antibiotics are used if indicated to increase comfort (e.g., in dysuria or cellulitis). As in Levels 1 through 3, tube feedings are used as needed.

*Level 5.* The patient receives supportive care and limited medical interventions, as defined in Level 4, and in addition is not given tube feeding by nasogastric tube or gastrostomy when normal food intake is no longer possible. Fluids for hydration are provided orally only if the patient is not comatose.

There is support for offering palliative choices to families of patients with DAT. For instance, the 1991 Congressional Advisory Panel on Alzheimer's Disease affirmed that the decision-making process "allow individualization of care and acceptance of some degree of risk in clinical and everyday care situations" (p. xxi).

At the abstract level, assigning patients to a level of care and carrying out the health care activities that emanate from those decisions is rather straightforward. In the clinical setting, at the operational level, such decisions that specify the level of technology to be applied or withheld are not related to hypothetical events that have a low possibility of occurring. Patients ultimately die from a complication of DAT or, more accurately stated, from the consequences of the natural progression of DAT.

Participation in the making and implementation of these decisions has profound effects on all. The patients who can no longer make or articulate a decision are dependent upon their surrogate decision makers to represent their wishes and upon the health care team to responsibly carry out those wishes. Patients' surrogates maintain the ethical principle of autonomy for patients but may carry an additional burden if they have selected comfort over maintaining life at all costs as they witness the symptoms of the relentless progression of DAT in their loved one. Clinicians are concerned with the ethical principle of beneficence/nonmaleficence. Because of their professional education and experience, clinicians are better prepared than surrogates or the courts for making and implementing decisions that pose ethical and clinical dilemmas. However, some clinicians, whose purpose in entering the health care field was the ability to cure and restore, now may be required to withhold therapy that could, at least in theory, extend life, in order to assure a comfortable death.

In the high-touch paradigm an interdisciplinary team approach to care with a focus on maintaining comfort is established and followed for all patients. Each patient has an individualized care plan that directs the application of professional and assisted services required, and a copy is sent to the family for their information and input.

The Advance Proxy Planning that determines medical technology to be applied if certain complications/consequences of DAT occur also establishes the foci for high-touch care. For each level of care, as a specific medical intervention is not applied, there are intensive care nursing interventions that are applied.

When a patient is assigned to Level 1, there is no directive to limit medical interventions, and intensive high-tech health care resources would be applied as necessary. The staff supports the family in their decision and do all in their power to maintain patient comfort despite the application of technology. If a patient must go to the x-ray department, a staff member would accompany the patient if at all possible. When transferred to an acute care unit, detailed verbal and written reports are provided to the new caregivers for communicating techniques that have been effective in providing direct care to the patient.

Patients assigned to Level 2 have a DNR order. The DNR decision no longer presents an ethical dilemma as clinicians recognize both the futility (Awoke, Mouton, & Parrott, 1992) and

adverse effects (Applebaum, King, & Finucane, 1990) of cardiopulmonary resuscitation on long-term care patients in general, and
its use is low (Duthie et al., 1993). Resuscitation for an unwitnessed
cardiac arrest in this population has a very low probability of
restoring life (Duthie et al., 1993). Patients who survive and are
discharged back to their long-term care unit are often in a more
advanced stage of dementia than they were before the arrest. A
DNR order would spare the few patients who survive the resuscitation event from living in an uncomfortable state for the remain-
der of their lives. If the definition of success is to restore patients
to their previous functional capacity, no matter how limited, then
there is no place for resuscitation attempts when patients with
DAT suffer from cardiac or respiratory arrest.

Level 3, not transferring patients to acute care units, presents
more of a dilemma. For instance, coronary bypass surgery might
extend the life of a patient who has severe coronary disease. On
the other hand, living on a long-term care unit without perceiv-
ing the stresses of the world and receiving care in a low-stimulus
environment may be clinically advantageous. Cataract surgery may
be advocated to allow patients the ability to connect visually with
their environment. However, patients will be at risk of removing
an intraocular lens because, unless restrained, they would be likely
to rub the eye. Regardless of the medical intervention, a transfer
to an acute care unit also means that patients will be cared for by
staff who may be experts in critical care but not in dementia care.
Transferring patients to acute units also predisposes them to trans-
location stress (Dehlin, 1990).

On acute care units there is an increased potential for the use
of restraints, which can predispose patients to increased delirium
and the complications of immobility. A vicious circle of events
leading to increased iatrogenesis can be set in motion. The issue
of the application of restraints to deliver technology the patient
cannot understand is complex. One could argue that the patient
will forget being restrained and the long-term benefit outweighs
the short-term requirement of being in restraints. On the other
hand, because patients with DAT appear to live in the present,
the stress associated with being restrained is not outweighed by
the ability to deliver technology. Patients with late-stage DAT have
a reduced life span, which needs to be considered when the question is asked: Is the burden outweighed by the benefit?

Level 4, not performing a complete diagnostic workup followed by aggressive management of intercurrent infections, appears on the surface to be denying patients lifesaving therapy that is relatively routine care. However, there is little specific information regarding treatment strategies for caring for DAT patients who develop intercurrent infections. This paucity of information exists despite the fact that patients with late-stage DAT develop risk factors that predispose them to infection. Incontinence places patients at risk of urinary tract infections (Lipsky, 1989; Parulkar & Barrett, 1988). Mobility and eating difficulties that predispose DAT patients to aspiration (Campbell-Taylor & Fisher, 1987; Knebl, Feinberg, & Tully, 1989) may cause pneumonia, which often has atypical clinical presentations (Andrews, Chandrasekaran, & McSwiggin, 1984; Finkelstein, Petkum, & Freedman, 1983; Harper & Newton, 1989).

An abundance of work related to nursing home infections and antibiotic use in the elderly was cited in the review articles of Magaziner et al. (1991) and Warren et al. (Warren, Palumbo, Fitterman, Speedie, 1991). However, these studies were from demographic and utilization perspectives and did not discuss any downside of aggressive treatment practices. Issues of increased discomfort or iatrogenesis associated with diagnosis or treatment (i.e., effects of withholding antipyretics until a fever spikes and a blood culture can be obtained or applying restraints so that intravenous antibiotics can be given) were not addressed.

Fabiszewski and colleagues have initiated the work to address the preceding issues. They have characterized the clinical trajectory of decline in patients with late-stage DAT who developed fevers (Fabiszewski et al., 1988) and examined the survival of patients treated aggressively and palliatively (Fabiszewski, Volicer, & Volicer, 1990). The latter study followed late-stage DAT patients during a 34-month evaluation period, in which 75 of 104 patients developed a total of 172 fever episodes. Patients were divided into four categories according to the severity of their DAT (very high vs. high) and treatment approach (palliative vs. aggressive treatment). There was no difference in survival for the two groups of patients with more severe DAT. The survival rate was lower for patients with less severe DAT who were treated palliatively than for those who were treated aggressively.

As a result, the investigators recommended that treatment decisions be made individually for each patient, which requires that both family and staff know the risks and benefits of different strategies. The aggressive treatment of infection does not affect the progressive and incurable nature of DAT. Treatment of infection(s) in patients with severe DAT may not affect overall mortality rates and could be considered futile (Fabiszewski et al., 1990). In the absence of achieving a long-term benefit, it might be more prudent to avoid future treatments that invoke patient discomfort and utilize health care resources for futile medical interventions.

A follow-up study (Hurley, Volicer, Mahoney, & Volicer, 1993) examined discomfort and health care resources utilized during fever episodes. Comparable patients were recruited and characterized, using similar scales. Discomfort was defined as a negative emotional and/or physical state, subject to variation in magnitude in response to internal or environmental conditions and operationalized by the Discomfort Scale for DAT (DS-DAT) (Hurley et al., 1992). The DS-DAT is a 9-item behavioral observation scale with a range of 0 (no observed discomfort) to 27 (high level of observed discomfort). The DS-DAT was administered monthly to all patients and during the typical peak (Days 3–5) and resolution (Days 9–11) for those who developed febrile episodes.

Observed discomfort levels before, at peak, and at resolution were higher for patients treated aggressively on traditional long-term care units than for patients cared for on special care dementia units. The burden associated with fever management strategies needs to be considered in the light of iatrogenesis and benefits. Most patients who develop fevers have multiple episodes and recover with or without using antibiotics, which can promote resistance, necessitating the administration of more potent parenteral antibiotics.

Level 4 makes operational the fact that there is no need for patients to endure invasive treatments that do not treat underlying causes when symptomatic management promoting comfort is more appropriate. Liberal antipyretics are used. Also, low oral doses of morphine by mouth are effective and should be considered as an analgesic treatment. Morphine has few side effects, and addiction to narcotics for patients with late-stage DAT is not an issue. The side effect of constipation is not an issue because we assume most patients develop constipation even without morphine in late-stage dementia, and therefore all patients receive special interventions to prevent impaction.

Patients assigned to Level 5 are fed by natural means even when they develop eating problems. The investigation of eating problems has been pursued actively at the Bedford VA Medical Center (Volicer, Fabiszweski, Rheaume, & Lasch, 1988). Clinical research has addressed the special nutritional needs of DAT patients (Rheaume, Riley, & Volicer, 1987), characteristics of eating difficulties (Volicer et al., 1989), special diets (Warden, 1989), and the use of dietary supplements (Riley & Volicer, 1990). Drawing on this expertise, Volicer, Rheaume, Riley, Karner, and Glennon (1990) demonstrated that it was possible to resume natural feeding in five of six DAT patients who had chronic feeding tubes.

One patient's story will be used to illustrate the clinical reasons for promoting natural versus artificial feeding. The patient had been admitted to the hospital because of resistive behaviors at home, having refused food and fluids. Because of the subsequent dehydration and lethargy, he was fed by a gastrostomy tube. Restraints were used to prevent the patient from removing the tube. When he was admitted to the DSCU, the family agreed to a trial of natural feeding. The patient was able to be fed successfully until his death 10 months later from complications of volvulus of the distal jejunum around peritoneal adhesions. This patient clearly had an improvement in quality of life by being able to taste food again and having increased caregiver interaction during feeding.

The Norberg studies (Athlin & Norberg, 1987a, 1987b; Michaelsson, Norberg, & Norberg, 1987; Norberg, Norberg, & Bexell, 1980) describe the importance, from both ethical and clinical perspectives, of interaction with demented patients during feeding. In some other settings, a feeding tube is regarded as a lifeline, and when staff plan to send a patient for a gastrostomy tube placement, they speak almost reverently. One is reminded of the early days of hemodialysis, when the placement of a shunt was indeed a lifeline. In this case, the question posed can be: Is the "lifeline" a substitute for the process of staff interaction when feeding a terminal patient? The suggested solution is to give small quantities of a liquid dietary formula by mouth, using slow and skillful feeding techniques.

Both staff and family need to be prepared for the time when patients will be unable to drink even water by mouth. Although palliative care clinicians (Billings, 1985; Cassem, 1985) advocate that dehydration is a natural painless antecedent to death, symbolism cannot be overlooked. Because of the emotional and nurturing significance of food and fluid, the issue of dying in a dehydrated state may be more of a problem to staff and families than to the patient. Brown and Hekryn (1989) consider the withdrawal from food made by terminally ill patients to be part of the body's process of preparing for death. Dying patients do not report the classical dehydration symptoms of headache, nausea, vomiting, or cramps (Billings, 1985). Thirst and dry mouth are the symptoms that bother patients (Billings, 1985), and these symptoms can be alleviated by intensive nursing care. Providing ice chips and frequent mouth care are advocated. A nursing staff member described this process "I would sit with him, and it was just one ice chip at a time."

In summary, when patients are allowed to receive palliative care, their families, as surrogate decision makers, have rejected high-tech care that can prolong the dying process. Instead, patients receive high-touch care provided by interdisciplinary health care team members who are all shareholders in a well-defined plan in which the goal is to provide patient comfort.

The paradigm of high-touch care provides intensive care nursing, rather than the medicalization of late-stage DAT. High-touch care is congruent with contemporary policy recommendations and biomedical ethics and involves the interdisciplinary team to promote mutual goal setting in collaboration with the family (Mahoney, Hurley, Smith, & Volicer, 1992). Patients' dignity and individuality, as remembered by the family and preserved by the staff, may be maintained despite the relentless progression of DAT.

## ACKNOWLEDGMENTS

The authors wish to thank the patients, families, and staff of the Edith Nourse Rogers Memorial Veterans Hospital, Bedford, Massachusetts, for their contributions to this chapter. The writing of this chapter was supported in part by a grant from the National Center of Nursing Research (R03NR02829) to A. Hurley and L. Volicer and by the Department of Veterans Affairs Gerontological Nurse Fellowship to M. Mahoney.

## REFERENCES

Advisory Panel on Alzheimer's Disease. (1991). *Second report of the advisory panel on Alzheimer's disease* (DHHS Publication No. ADM91-1791). Washington, DC: U.S. Government Printing Office.

Andrews, J., Chandrasekaran, P., & McSwiggin, D. (1984). Lower respiratory tract infections in an acute geriatric male ward: One-year prospective surveillance. *Gerontology, 30,* 290–292.

Applebaum, G. E., King, J. E., & Finucane, T. E. (1990). The outcome of cardiopulmonary resuscitation initiated in nursing homes. *Journal of the American Geriatrics Society, 38,* 197–200.

Athlin, E., & Norberg, A. (1987a). Caregivers' attitudes to and interpretations of the behavior of severely demented patients during feeding in a patient assignment care system. *International Journal of Nursing Studies, 24,* 145–153.

Athlin, E., & Norberg, A. (1987b). Interaction between the demented patient and his caregiver during feeding. *Scandinavian Journal of the Caring Sciences, 1,* 117–122.

Awoke, S., Mouton, C., & Parrott, M. (1992). Outcomes of skilled cardiopulmonary resuscitation in a long-term care facility: Futile therapy? *Journal of the American Geriatrics Society, 40,* 593–595.

Billings, J. A. (1985). Comfort measures for the terminally ill. *Journal of the American Geriatrics Society, 33,* 808–810.

Brown, P., & Hekryn, J. (1989). The dying patient and dehydration. *Canadian Nurse, 85,* 14–16.

Campbell-Taylor, I., & Fisher, R. H. (1987). The clinical case against tube feeding in palliative care of the elderly. *Journal of the American Geriatrics Society, 35,* 1100–1104.

Cassem, N. H. (1980). Appropriate treatment limits in advanced cancer. In J. Billings (Ed.), *Outpatient management of advance cancer: Symptom control, support and hospice-in-the-home.* Philadelphia: J. B. Lippincott.

Dehlin, O. (1990). Relocation of patients with senile dementia: Effects on symptoms and mortality. *Journal of Clinical and Experimental Gerontology, 12,* 1–12.

Duthie, E., Mark, D., Tresch, D., Kartes, S., Neahring, J., & Aufderheide, T. (1993). Utilization of cardiopulmonary resuscitation in nursing homes in one community: Rates and nursing home characteristics. *Journal of the American Geriatrics Society, 41,* 384–388.

Fabiszewski, K. J., Riley, M. E., Berkley, D., Karner, J., & Shea, S. (1988). Management of advanced Alzheimer dementia. In L. Volicer, K. J. Fabiszewski, Y. L. Rheaume, & K. E. Lasch (Eds.)., *Clinical manage-*

*ment of Alzheimer's disease* (pp. 87-109). Rockville, MD, Royal Tunbridge Wells: Aspen.

Fabiszewski, K. J., Volicer, B., & Volicer, L. (1990). Effect of antibiotic treatment on outcome of fevers in institutionalized Alzheimer patients. *Journal of the American Medical Association, 263,* 3168-3172.

Finkelstein, M. S., Petkum, W. M., & Freedman, M. L. (1983). Pneumococcal bacteremia in adults: Age-dependent differences in presentation and in outcome. *Journal of the American Geriatrics Society, 31,* 19-27.

Harper, C., & Newton, P. (1989). Clinical aspects of pneumonia in the elderly veteran. *Journal of the American Geriatrics Society, 37,* 867-872.

Hurley, A. C., Volicer, B. J., Hanrahan, P., Houde, S., & Volicer, L. (1992). Assessment of discomfort in advanced Alzheimer patients. *Research in Nursing and Health, 15,* 369-377.

Hurley, A. C., Volicer, B. J., Mahoney, M. A., & Volicer, L. (1993). Palliative fever management in Alzheimer patients: Quality plus fiscal responsibility. *Advances in Nursing Science, 16*(1).

Knebl, J., Feinberg, M., & Tully, J. (1989). The relationship of pneumonia and aspiration in an elderly population. *Gerontologist, 29,* 195A.

Lipsky, B. A. (1989). Urinary tract infections in men: Epidemiology, pathophysiology, diagnosis, and treatment. *Annals of Internal Medicine, 110,* 138-150.

Maas, M. (1988). Management of patients with Alzheimer's disease in long-term care facilities. In I. L. Abraham, K. C. Buckwalter, & M. M. Neundorfer (Eds.), *The nursing clinics of North America* (pp. 57-68). Philadelphia: W. B. Saunders.

Magaziner, J., Tenney, J. H., DeForge, B., Hebel, R., Munice, H. L., & Warren, J. W. (1991). Prevalence and characteristics of nursing home-acquired infections in the aged. *Journal of the American Geriatrics Society, 39,* 1071-1078.

Mahoney, M. A., Hurley, A., Smith, S., & Volicer, L. (1992). Advance management preferences: The nurse's role in surrogate decision making about life sustaining interventions. In G. B. White (Ed.), *Ethical dilemmas in nursing practice* (pp. 45-58). Kansas City, MO: American Nurses Association.

Michaelsson, E., Norberg, A., & Norberg, B. (1987). Feeding methods for demented patients in end stage of life. *Geriatric Nursing, 8,* 69-73.

Norberg, A., Norberg, B., & Bexell, G. (1980). Ethical problems in feeding patients with advanced dementia. *British Medical Journal, 281,* 847-848.

Parulkar, B. J., & Barrett, D. M. (1988). Urinary incontinence in adults. *Surgical Clinics of North America, 68,* 945–963.

Rheaume, Y., Riley, M. E., & Volicer, L. (1987). Meeting nutritional needs of Alzheimer patients who pace constantly. *Journal of Nutrition of the Elderly, 7,* 43–52.

Riley, M. E. & Volicer, L. (1990). Evaluation of a new nutritional supplement for patients with Alzheimer's disease. *Journal of the American Dietetic Association, 90,* 433–435.

Robinson, B. E., Sucholeiki, R., & Schocken, D. D. (1993). Sudden death and resisted mechanical restraint: A case report. *Journal of the American Geriatrics Society, 41,* 424–425.

U.S. Congress, Office of Technology Assessment. (1990). *Confused minds, burdened families: Finding help for people with Alzheimer's and other dementias.* Washington, DC: U.S. Government Printing Office.

Volicer, L. (1986). Need for hospice approach to treatment of patients with advanced progressive dementia. *Journal of the American Geriatrics Society, 34,* 655–658.

Volicer, L., & Fabiszewski, K. J. (1988). The use of medical technology in advanced Alzheimer disease. *American Journal of Alzheimer's Care and Related Disorders and Research, 3,* 11–17.

Volicer, L., Fabiszewski, K. J., Rheaume, Y. L., & Lasch, K. E. (1988). *Clinical management of Alzheimer's disease.* Rockville, MD, Royal Tunbridge Wells: Aspen.

Volicer, L., Rheaume, Y., Brown, J., Fabiszewski, K., & Brady, R. (1986). Hospice approach to the treatment of patients with advanced dementia of the Alzheimer type. *Journal of the American Medical Association, 256,* 2210–2213.

Volicer, L., Rheaume, Y., Riley, M. E., Karner, J., & Glennon, M. (1990). Discontinuation of tube feeding in patients with dementia of the Alzheimer type. *American Journal of Alzheimer's Care and Related Disorders and Research, 5,* 22–25.

Volicer, L., Seltzer, B., Rheaume, Y., Fabiszewski, K., Herz, L., Shapiro, R., & Innis, P. (1987). Progression of Alzheimer-type dementia in institutionalized patients: A cross-sectional study. *Journal of Applied Gerontology, 6,* 83–94.

Volicer, L., Seltzer, B., Rheaume, Y., Karner, J., Glennon, M., Riley, M. E., & Crino, P. B. (1989). Eating difficulties in patients with probable dementia of the Alzheimer's type. *Journal of Geriatric Psychiatry and Neurology, 2,* 169–176.

Warden, V. J. (1989). Waste not, want not. *Geriatric Nursing, 10,* 210–211.

Warren, J. W., Palumbo, F. B., Fitterman, L., & Speedie, S. M. (1991). Incidence and characteristics of antibiotic use in aged nursing home patients. *Journal of the American Geriatrics Society, 39*, 963–972.

## THE CASE OF MS. F

Ms. F is a blind 92-year-old woman who has resided in your nursing home for about 1 year. Ms. F had suffered from severe arthritis, which left her markedly incapacitated physically but still able to communicate. Ms. F has one child, a very devoted son.

Several months after his mother entered your facility, Ms. F's son approaches you and says that he knows his mother would not want her life prolonged should her condition worsen in any way. Although she is unable to see and is extremely hard of hearing, Ms. F is still able to communicate with you. Therefore, you approach her and ask if she would like to discuss her treatment preferences in the event she becomes unable to do so. She agrees to this and with you, her son, and her social worker in attendance executes a health care proxy in which she names her son as agent.

Several months later, Ms. F suffers a stroke and is unable to communicate and unable to eat. Her physicians feel strongly that she has no hope of recovery, and it is obvious that she cannot make treatment decisions for herself at this time. Accordingly, her son begins to act as her health care agent.

Because she is not eating or drinking, an IV is started. After several days of IV therapy, the primary care team responsible for Ms. F's care contemplates the insertion of a feeding tube. When they discuss this with Ms. F's son, he tells you that he and his mother have often discussed issues around life prolongation and that she had voiced a particular repugnance to the idea of being fed via a tube. Therefore, he asks you not to insert a feeding tube and also to remove the IV and let his mother die in peace. Because it is obvious that she will not recover and because he is her legal agent for health care decisions, you and his primary health care team tell him you will abide by his—and his mother's— wishes with respect to treatment.

Periodically, a staff member enters her room and moistens her lips. A comfort care regimen, including mouth care, is instituted. Approximately every 2 hours, the staff turns and positions Ms. F. Most of the time, her son is in attendance and needs frequent reassurance from the staff that his mother is comfortable.

When it appears that death will probably occur within the next few days, Ms. F's son decides to remain at her bedside around the clock. Ms. F begins to moan when she is turned and positioned. She also breathes heavily and sounds congested. Her son is concerned that she is in pain and requests something to stop the moaning. The staff wishes to suction Ms. F because they feel her discomfort is related to her chest congestion. The son refuses to let them do so, stating that it is too invasive a procedure for a dying patient. Small doses of morphine are ordered, to be given as needed, but Ms. F's son complains that the nurses seem reluctant to give it, disagreeing with the son that his mother is in pain.

## QUESTIONS FOR DISCUSSION

1. Why is it important to attempt to ascertain whether Ms. F could indicate her own treatment preferences?
2. Why is it important to determine that there is no hope of recovery?
3. Why do you think the nurses might be reluctant to give the morphine? What strategies might be employed to assist them?
4. In addition to mouth care, turning and positioning, and administering pain medication to Ms. F, is there anything else that the staff could or should do to assist her through the dying process?
5. What should be done to support Ms. F's son?

## ANSWERS

Too frequently, older people, particularly those who are exceedingly frail or have seemingly limited cognitive ability, are assumed to be totally unable to make their wishes known. However, very often skillful questioning will elicit appropriate responses to queries about whom they would like to make decisions for them or if they would want to be fed via a tube should they become unable to eat. And given the prominence of patient autonomy in current practice, it is important that every person have the right to make his or her wishes known. Accordingly, as noted in several of the other cases, even when the person made his or her treatment preferences known at some earlier time, he or she should be consulted again if at all possible when determining the course of action regarding treatment.

Additionally, as noted elsewhere (see "The Case of Ms. C" pp. 38–42, this volume), many conditions that are potentially life-threatening in older people are reversible and if properly diagnosed and treated, can be resolved. Accordingly, before considering limiting life-sustaining treatment, it is important to ascertain whether Ms. F's condition indeed cannot be treated and reversed.

When it comes to pain medication for patients very near the end of life, physicians and nurses are often concerned that the administration of this medication may "push the patient over the edge." Nurses in particular, who are usually responsible for the actual administration of the drug, may feel that they actually "caused" the patient's death.

Nurses and physicians working in these situations clearly need emotional support. Perhaps more important, however, they need to be educated about the ethical principle of "double effect" and reminded that acceptable practice—legal, medical, and ethical—permits the use of potent analgesics to relieve pain at the end of life even if their administration causes death to occur sooner than it might have otherwise. They should also be educated regarding other forms of discomfort, such as dyspnea, that are common symptoms in terminal illness and reminded that it is acceptable to administer drugs like morphine for relief. Oxygen may also be useful, as well as anticholinergic agents such as scopolamine, if there is chest congestion (Cooke, 1989; Saunders, 1982).

The nursing staff should receive extensive education in the provision of comfort care. The administration of pain medication, regular turning and positioning, and very frequent mouth care should be routine when caring for someone dying after life-sustaining treatment has been withheld or withdrawn. In addition, the nursing staff and other staff members involved with the care of Ms. F should be encouraged to continue to talk to Ms. F, hold her hand, and touch her frequently. This may be as beneficial to the staff as it is to Ms. F because it will remind them that they are not abandoning her but continuing to provide the same (if not even higher) level of caring as Ms. F nears death as they did while she was very much alive.

Anecdotal evidence suggests that, even when health care agents are convinced they are carrying out the wishes of the person who named them as agents, making a decision to limit life-sustaining treatment is exceedingly difficult and emotionally wrenching. Thus, the provision of comfort care to Ms. F—through both physical and emotional means—will, by extension, be comforting to Ms. F's son. In addition, time must be spent with Ms. F's son, reassuring him that not only did he follow his mother's wishes, but that those wishes are being carried out in the most compassionate manner. Family members of dying patients have a need to feel accepted and supported by health professionals, and they report deriving comfort when those who are caring for the dying person also offer solace to families (Hampe, 1976).

## REFERENCES

Cooke, N. (1989). Dyspnea. In T. D. Walsh (Ed.), *Symptom control.* Boston: Blackwell Scientific Publications.

Hampe, S. O. (1976). Needs of the grieving spouse in a hospital setting. *Nursing research, 24,* 113–120.

Saunders, C. (1982). Principles of symptom control in terminal care. *Medical Clinics of North America, 66,* 1169–83.

# 7

# The Role of Antibiotics in Comfort Care

*Jack P. Freer and*
*David W. Bentley*

The provision of comfort care is the most important treatment option we can offer to dying patients who are beyond cure. When we can no longer cure or ensure long-term survival, palliative treatments are still available and grow in importance. Furthermore, when a conscious decision to forgo life-sustaining therapy is made, the goals and objectives of medical treatment change in dramatic fashion. Further survival becomes unimportant or even undesirable; comfort and peace of mind become paramount.

A variety of medical interventions have been adapted for use in comfort care. Most notably, narcotics and other analgesics have broad applicability in relieving the distress of the dying patient. No longer limited to pain control, their use has been expanded selectively to include sedation or relief of dyspnea. Such uses have sharpened the focus on the role these drugs play in hastening the death of some patients. A consensus is evolving that holds that such treatments, in carefully chosen situations, are justifiable when used for symptom control, even if they contribute to the patient's demise (Edwards & Ueno, 1991).

A comprehensive palliative care plan must take advantage of the full therapeutic armamentarium available to the clinician. This chapter will discuss one specific therapeutic agent, namely, antibiotics. To help focus this discussion, several questions will be posed: What is "comfort care"? Are the usual outcomes of antibiotic treatment consistent with the goals of comfort care? When does the use of antibiotics constitute comfort care? What are the frequent infections afflicting end-stage dementia patients that are likely to contribute to their suffering? When are antibiotics more likely to be burdensome? We conclude with a discussion of how a flexible approach to comfort care, including the use of antibiotics, can result in enhanced symptomatic relief for the dying patient.

## CONCEPTUAL FRAMEWORK

It should first be noted that the approach presented here is predicated upon certain ethical and legal presumptions. For the purpose of our discussion, we will assume that patient autonomy is held paramount. In holding to accepted standards, competent patients must be given maximum freedom to participate in the decision-making process (Beauchamp & Childress, 1989). When patients lose decision-making capacity, appropriate means to protect autonomy (including advance directives) are assumed to guide treatment decisions (Buchanan & Brock, 1989); (President's Commission, 1983). Clearly, the approaches to curative versus palliative care may differ when the above-noted presumptions are not valid. The fact remains, in most situations of end-stage dementia, the clinician and family are faced with painful decisions.

Many therapeutic interventions have the potential to extend life. Under usual circumstances, we properly assume that sustaining life is an appropriate goal of medical treatment. We therefore have the obligation to provide such treatment or justify the decision to forgo such therapy. In recent years, there has been much written about these decisions and the evolving consensus they have generated (Meisel, 1992; Veatch, 1993).

Traditionally, therapies are assessed in terms of their burdens and benefits. If a treatment's burden outweighs its benefit (from the patient's perspective), it should not be provided unless the patient accepts that burden. It has become clear, however, that some simpler, less invasive therapies may also be withheld using this rubric. In cases where quality of life is so poor that life itself is not worth living, any treatment that extends life (no matter how simple) is potentially more burden than benefit (Paris, 1986). It is therefore quite appropriate to permit a liberal and individualized interpretation of "burden of treatment." This is clearly in keeping with the principle of autonomy by which each patient personally decides which outcomes are desirable and which are undesirable.

Specifically excluded from this discussion are the concepts of ordinary/extraordinary therapy, natural death/death with dignity, and prolongation of the dying process. Although these slogans have popular appeal, they are imprecise and generally not helpful in problem solving. The framework we have outlined above will be sufficient to address the questions and added dilemmas raised by the use of antibiotics as comfort care.

## COMFORT CARE

What is comfort care? Implicit in any discussion of comfort care is the notion that such therapy is somehow different from curative treatment that also provides symptomatic relief. Many therapies provide comfort and relieve symptoms in addition to extending life. This seems not to be what most people would consider comfort care. One therefore might interpret comfort care as "comfort care only."

In reality, however, all treatment modalities have a multidimensional profile of characteristics and have varying degrees of efficacy at producing certain responses. A graphic display is useful in portraying these issues. In Figure 7.1, quality of life (i.e., the presence or absence of pain and suffering) is plotted against quantity of life (i.e., added months of living). Region E is the baseline untreated state. It represents the natural history of the patient's disease when untreated. Regions A, B, and C are the result of effective symptomatic treatment, but only treatment categorized as A and B would be considered comfort care or comfort care only. Region A, however, is palliative care that hastens death (such as narcotics for terminal pain or to relieve dyspnea).

Regions C, F, and I represent what we have characterized as life-sustaining treatments. Region C is typically identified with ideal therapy: that which prolongs life and provides symptom relief. This is, of course, not ideal therapy in those situations alluded to above in which continued life itself is a burden.

Certainly, it is expeditious to categorize treatment as comfort care or life-sustaining. In real life, however, treatments not only

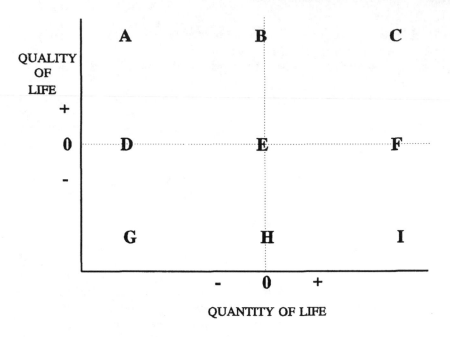

**Figure 7.1.** Multidimensional profile of treatment modalities. The characterization of treatment options is based upon their ability to influence survival and suffering and includes Region A: treatment that is likely to relieve suffering but shorten survival; Region B: treatment that is likely to relieve suffering, with no effect on survival; Region C: treatment that is likely to relieve suffering and prolong survival; Region D: treatment that is likely to shorten survival, with no effect on suffering; Region E: the expected clinical course without treatment or with treatment that has no effect on either survival or suffering; Region F: treatment that is likely to prolong survival, with no effect on suffering; Region G: treatment that is likely to worsen suffering and shorten survival; Region H: treatment that is likely to worsen suffering, with no effect on survival; Region I: treatment that is likely to prolong survival but worsen suffering.

have positive features of both but also may have negative features as well. For example, palliative treatments may shorten survival (A), and life-sustaining treatments may diminish quality of life (I).

## ANTIBIOTICS AS COMFORT CARE

Antibiotic therapy can be categorized as life-sustaining treatment. Although not typically included among the more dramatic interventions (such as CPR or mechanical ventilation), it has been recognized as lifesaving in many situations (Bentley et al., 1986; U.S. Congress, 1987). Thus, choosing to forgo antibiotics is characterized as a grave decision that would hasten a patient's death (Brown & Thompson, 1979; Hilfiker, 1983; Wanzer et al., 1984). This presumption is not valid, however, for the severely demented in long-term settings, for whom nontreatment may result in similar survival when compared to those treated with antibiotics (Fabiszewski, Volicer, & Volicer, 1990). Regardless of their effectiveness, attention has always been focused upon antibiotics' potential to prolong life. There has been little attention, however, to the role of antibiotics as comfort care. Otherwise exhaustive manuals of palliative care often contain no mention of antibiotics (University of Toronto, 1989).

Are the usual outcomes of antibiotic therapy consistent with the goals of comfort care? To answer this we must broaden the focus on our definition of comfort care. As noted earlier, some therapies are strictly comfort measures only because they offer no hope of cure or long-term survival. Simple analgesics fall into this category. Treatments described as comfort care only can be placed in regions A and B in Figure 7.1.

We are left, however, with the dilemma of how to characterize Region C. Although potentially offering excellent symptom relief, these therapies are not usually considered palliative because they also cure and extend life. In fact, antibiotics (if effective), are certain to be found somewhere in Region C. This is because the symptomatic relief produced by antibiotics is closely linked to its life-sustaining properties. Because antibiotic therapy relieves symptoms by its antimicrobial actions, antibiotics relieve symptoms to the degree that they have the potential to cure. Antibiotic therapy is therefore rarely found in the regions identified as comfort care only (A and B). Certain antibiotics may fail to cure infections, but they would also fail to relieve symptoms in such cases.

When does the use of antibiotics constitute comfort care? To designate antibiotic treatment as comfort care, we must broaden the scope of our definition of antibiotic effectiveness. We would suggest that antibiotic therapy is comfort care when it is uniquely effective at relieving symptoms. That is to say, antibiotics relieve symptoms in ways that no other therapy can. This derives both from the specificity of the therapy and the side effects of alternative treatment options.

In the examples provided below, note that some symptoms associated with infections are relieved uniquely by antibiotics. Alternative palliative treatments often include high doses of analgesics or sedatives with obvious side effects. Although in this setting antibiotics are considered comfort care, it does not necessarily mandate their use. Patients (or surrogates) must still decide on which course of action is preferable. In a later section, we will offer guidance in making such decisions.

## EXAMPLES

What are the frequent infections afflicting end-stage dementia patients that are likely to contribute to their suffering? These patients are often bedridden, malnourished, and incontinent, often with chronic indwelling bladder (Foley) catheters. Furthermore, coexisting illnesses may also compromise the elderly demented patient's ability to deal with infection. Residents in long-term care facilities (LTCFs) have the additional problem of drug-resistant organisms that commonly cause nosocomial infections (Beam, 1989; U. S. Congress, 1987).

The three most frequent life-threatening infections identified by the report *Life Sustaining Technologies and the Elderly* (U.S. Congress, 1987) include pneumonia, urinary tract infection, and infected pressure sores. These are also the most common serious infections in LCTFs. These examples will demonstrate how the flexible approach to decision making we propose is well suited to the problem of infection in end-stage dementia patients residing in LTCFs. Furthermore, they will illustrate how optimal palliative care is achieved when an antibiotic's unique effectiveness is weighed against its potential to prolong life, in light of alternative comfort measures.

In general, any of these infections can produce nonspecific as well as disease-specific symptoms. The nonspecific symptoms include fever, chills, anorexia, malaise, falls, confusion, and recent-onset incontinence (Rosenthal & Steel, 1990). The disease-specific symptoms are directly related to the site of infection, as noted below.

Pneumonia is the second most frequent cause of LTCF-acquired infection and is the leading cause of hospitalization and death in this high-risk population. Although pneumonia commonly presents with nonspecific symptoms, disease-specific symptoms and signs soon predominate (Bentley, 1988). Cough may be persistent and annoying and keep the patient awake. If productive, the sputum can be especially bothersome to patient and family alike if purulent, bloody, or malodorous. There may be significant pain if pleurisy is present. Severe dyspnea may be a significant problem as the disease progresses, either untreated or when resistant to therapy. This focal, disease-specific symptom could be relieved by the use of narcotics but would be associated with sedation.

The choice of treatment is thus narrowed to narcotics versus antibiotics with $O_2$ given in either case. We can predict that if effective, the antibiotic will provide relief from disease-specific and nonspecific symptoms. If ineffective, it will do nothing for either. The disease-specific effectiveness may well prove unique because it would permit a more alert state. This would presumably be desirable if the premorbid state was such that some aspects of life could still be enjoyed. The nonspecific relief offered by narcotics would presumably be less desirable in such a state.

We can identify these options on Figure 7.2. *X* represents palliative (narcotic) therapy only, *Y* represents ineffective antibiotic treatment, and *Z* represents effective antibiotic treatment. The latter offers a uniquely effective therapy that is indicated by its greater potential for enhancing quality of life (by reducing and eventually eliminating dyspnea, cough with purulent sputum, and pleurisy) than would the palliative alternative of $O_2$ and narcotics, which would likely require heavy sedation to give comparable relief. Note, however, that antibiotic treatment is in Region C in that it also prolongs life. As noted by Brown and Thompson (1979), mortality in nursing home residents can be reduced from 80% in untreated patients to 12% in antibiotic-treated patients. If the prepneumonia status of the patient was so wretched that pneumonia is a welcome mode of exit, then the "burden" of life prolongation would seem not to be worth the unique benefit the antibiotic would provide.

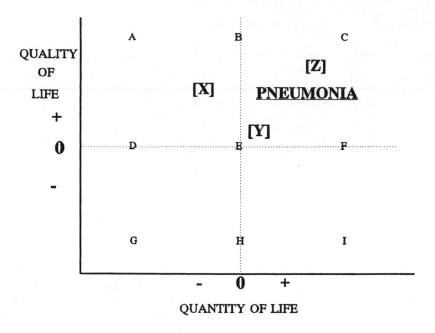

**Figure 7.2.** Treatment options for pneumonia occurring in end-stage dementia patients. *X* represents palliative therapy (narcotics, oxygen, etc.) only, *Y* represents ineffective antibiotic treatment, and *Z* represents effective antibiotic treatment. See Figure 7.1 for identification of regions A–I.

Urinary tract infections (UTIs) are the most frequent type of infection in the elderly. Most UTIs are asymptomatic and should not be treated with antibiotics (Bentley et al., 1986). When symptomatic, however, UTIs frequently cause irritative symptoms of dysuria, frequency, and nocturia, as well as new or worsening incontinence, gross hematuria, and flank pain (Nicolle, 1993). In these patients, antibiotics have an excellent chance of producing sustained symptomatic relief. If the predominant symptomatology results from septicemia, antibiotics are also effective (Brown & Thompson, 1979). But these patients also could be effectively treated nonspecifically if the premorbid quality of life is so poor that further survival is a burden.

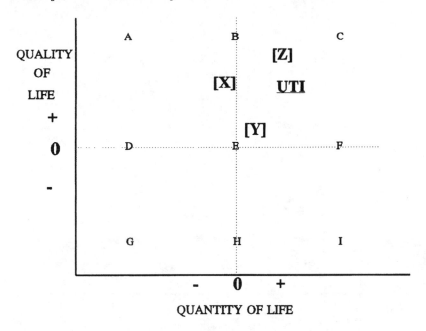

**Figure 7.3.** Treatment options for urinary tract infections occurring in end-stage dementia patients. *X* represents palliative therapy (narcotics, etc.) only, *Y* represents ineffective antibiotic treatment, and *Z* represents effective antibiotic treatment. See Figure 7.1 for identification of regions A–I.

Figure 7.3 illustrates the three treatment options for UTIs. Unlike narcotic use in pneumonia, its use in UTI is unlikely to hasten death. *X* is therefore closer to the "zero line" for quantity of life. *Z* is also closer to the zero line because untreated UTI is less likely to be life-threatening than pneumonia, and therefore antibiotics will be less life-sustaining. However, they can greatly enhance quality of life (Regions B and C).

Pressure (decubitus) ulcers occur frequently in residents of LTCFs. Resulting from immobility and excessive pressure and compounded by incontinence and malnutrition, ulcers are difficult to prevent in end-stage dementia patients and even more difficult to heal. Whereas ulcers frequently become infected (U.S. Congress, 1987), antibiotic treatment is but one small part of

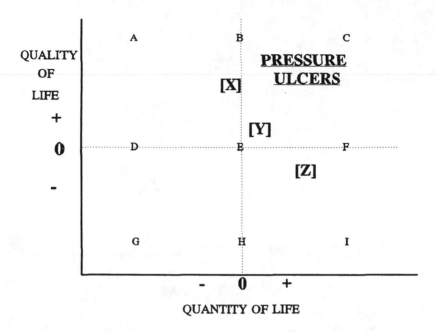

**Figure 7.4.** Treatment options for pressure (decubitus) ulcers occurring in end-stage dementia patients. *X* represents palliative therapy (narcotics) only, *Y* represents ineffective antibiotic treatment, and *Z* represents effective antibiotic treatment. See Figure 7.1 for identification of regions A–I.

aggressive attempts at healing such ulcers. Frequent repositioning to relieve excess pressure, nutritional support, and local wound care are all necessary. Even so, the infected ulcer may prove refractory to treatment and progress from Stage 3 to septicemia or to Stage 4, with osteomyelitis and death (Siegler & Lavizzo-Mourey, 1991).

The pain or discomfort of an infected pressure ulcer is often aggravated initially by local treatment. But unless local treatment (including removal of necrotic tissue, disinfection of the ulcer site, and dressings) is provided, the effectiveness of antibiotics will be limited. In fact, antibiotics are often reserved for the presence of cellulitis or suspected septicemia (Seiler & Stahelin, 1985). Therefore, the illustration for pressure ulcers (Figure 7.4) identifies the effective treatment as Option *Z* in Region I because of the likely burden that local treatment would necessitate to maximize the effectiveness of antibiotics. Antibiotics without local treatment (ineffective except for cellulitis) would probably be closer to $Y$. As with UTI, nonspecific palliative treatment $X$ is Region B.


## ANTIBIOTICS AS BURDENSOME TREATMENT

When are antibiotics more likely to be burdensome? In the discussion of antibiotics as comfort care, it was noted that if antibiotic use is effective, it would likely provide symptomatic relief to the same degree that it was life-sustaining. Admittedly, some organisms are resistant to certain antibiotics, and some infections are so overwhelming that antibiotic therapy is ineffective. In such cases, however, the antibiotic will not provide symptomatic relief either.

This is important in those patients for whom the quality of life is so poor that continued existence is undesirable. For such patients, any treatment with the potential to prolong life is a burden. Other circumstances in which antibiotics are burdensome include (1) whenever intravenous antibiotics are used, especially when they require hospitalization or restraints, and (2) when intramuscular antibiotics provide excess discomfort/pain or sterile abscesses. Most important, antibiotics are burdensome whenever cure of infection does not match the treatment goals of the demented patient.


## CONCLUSION

Providing comprehensive medical care to severely demented elderly residents in LTCFs or their homes is in many ways more difficult than in the usual situations, where the goal is always to prolong life. Any available treatment option has the potential to either enhance or diminish the quality of a patient's life. Similarly, that therapy might simultaneously prolong or shorten the patient's life. The ultimate decision to either provide or forgo the therapy must incorporate available information concerning the likely response to treatment and also reflect the patient's own values. This is best accomplished by means of a flexible approach that weighs all treatment options, together with the individual patient's attitudes and wishes.

This flexibility is important when treatment options appear to run counter to established practices and standards of care. The openness to utilizing treatment modalities in new ways has resulted in an evolution of thinking in the care of such patients. This maturation of thought is most evident in the "second look" of Wanzer and coworkers (1989). Whereas the earlier report (Wanzer et al., 1984) largely dealt with decisions to forgo the sustaining treatments, the later communication stressed the flexible approach in its recommendations to maximize symptom relief and even hasten death in some patients.

The flexible approach applied to antibiotic use is as follows. First, ask about the patient's premorbid quality of life. If acceptable, then antibiotics may offer a possibility of unique benefit, not achievable by narcotics or other nonspecific treatment. This would vary with the infection. UTIs and cellulitis, as we have seen, are most likely to be amenable to unique effects of antibiotics. Pneumonia is often amenable to antibiotic treatment even if attempts at drainage of respiratory secretions are less than optimal. Infected pressure ulcers are the most problematic for effective treatment if antibiotics alone are instituted without local wound care. In this case nonspecific treatment may be equally palliative.

Although further life is not the primary goal, it may be an acceptable side effect in order to gain symptomatic relief. If, however, the premorbid state is such that death is welcome, the burden that extended life carries makes it unacceptable. Simple narcotic therapy is then chosen. Finally, it is important to recognize that antibiotics are not uniformly effective.

Ultimately, the questions raised by this discussion of several key infections are more important than the specific comments we have offered. As long as clinicians remain flexible in their approach to comfort care, patients will be well served. Incorporation of antibiotic therapy into a palliative care plan that uses more traditional comfort measures (such as narcotics) can prove beneficial to hopelessly ill long-term care patients. Such patients and their families require skilled guidance in approaching these treatment decisions if patient comfort is to be maximized. Toward this end, any and all classes of drugs should be considered for use in comfort care.

## ACKNOWLEDGMENTS

We wish to acknowledge the helpful personal communications from Amanda Beck, MD, and the secretarial assistance of Rosemarie Cieslak and Arlene Peters.

## REFERENCES

Beam, T. R. (1989). Infections among nursing home residents: Preventive measures, diagnoses, and treatment options. In P. R. Katz & E. Calkins, (Eds.), *Principles and practice of nursing home care.* New York: Springer Publishing.

Beauchamp, T. L., & Childress, J. F. (1989). *Principles of biomedical ethics.* New York: Oxford University Press.

Bentley, D. W. (1988). Bacterial pneumonia in the elderly. *Hospital Practice, 23*(12), 99-116.

Bentley, D. W., Barker, W. H., Hunter, K. M., Mott, P. D., Phelps, C. E., & Takloski, P. A. (1986). *Antibiotics and the elderly.* Materials prepared for the U.S. Congress, Office of Technology Assessment, Washington, DC: U.S. Government Printing Office.

Brown, N. K., & Thompson, D. J. (1979). Nontreatment of fever in extended care facilities. *New England Journal of Medicine, 300,* 1246-1250.

Buchanan, A. E., & Brock, D. S. (1989). *Deciding for others: The ethics of surrogate decision making.* New York: Cambridge University Press.

Edwards, B. S., & Ueno, W. M. (1991). Sedation before ventilator withdrawal. *Journal of Clinical Ethics, 2,* 118-122.

Fabiszewski, K. J., Volicer, B., & Volicer, L. (1990). Effect of antibiotic treatment on outcome of fevers in institutionalized Alzheimer patients. *Journal of the American Medical Association, 263,* 3168-3172.

Hilfiker, D. (1983). Allowing the debilitated to die: Facing our ethical choices [Sounding Board]. *New England Journal of Medicine, 308,* 716-719.

Meisel, A. (1992). The legal consensus about forgoing life-sustaining treatment: Its status and its prospects. *Kennedy Institute of Ethics Journal, 2,* 309-345.

Nicolle, L. E. (1993). Urinary tract infections in long-term care facilities. *Infection Control and Hospital Epidemiology, 14,* 220-225.

Paris, J. J. (1986). When burdens of feeding outweigh benefits. *Hastings Center Report, 16*(1), 30-32.

President's Commission for the Study of Ethical Problems in Medicine and Biomedical and Behavioral Research. (1983). *Deciding to forego life-sustaining treatment: Ethical, medical and legal issues in treatment decisions*. Washington, DC: U.S. Government Printing Office.

Richardson, J. P. (1993). Bacteremia in the elderly. *Journal of General Internal Medicine, 8*, 89–92.

Rosenthal, G., & Steel, K. (1990). Differences in the presentation of disease. In W. R. Hazzard, R. Andres, E. L. Bierman, & J. P. Blass, (Eds.), *Principles of geriatric medicine and gerontology*. New York: McGraw-Hill.

Seiler, W. O., & Stahelin, H. B. (1985). Decubitus ulcers: Treatment through five therapeutic principles. *Geriatrics, 40*(9), 30–42.

Siegler, E. L., & Lavizzo-Mourey, R. (1991). Management of stage III pressure ulcers in moderately demented nursing home residents. *Journal of General Internal Medicine, 6*, 507–513.

University of Toronto, Sunnybrook Medical Centre. (1989). *Palliative care manual*. Toronto: Author.

U.S. Congress, Office of Technology Assessment. (1987). *Life-sustaining technologies and the elderly*. Washington, DC: U.S. Government Printing Office.

Veatch, R. M. (1993). Forgoing life-sustaining treatment: Limits to the consensus. *Kennedy Institute Ethics Journal, 3*, 1–19.

Wanzer, S. H., Adelstein, S. J., Cranford, R. E., Federman, D. D., Hook, E. D., Moertel, C. G., Safar, P., Stone, A., Taussig, H. B., & Eys, J. (1984). The physician's responsibility toward hopelessly ill patients. *New England Journal of Medicine, 310*, 955–959.

Wanzer, S. H., Federman, D. D., Adelstein, S. J., Cassel, C. K., Cassem, E. H., Cranford, R. E., Hook, E. W., Lo, B., Moertel, C. G., Safar, P., Stone, A., & Van Eys, J. (1989). The physician's responsibility toward hopelessly ill patients: A second look. *New England Journal of Medicine, 320*, 844–849.

## THE CASE OF MS. G

Ms. G, age 84, has been a resident in your nursing home for several years. A few weeks ago, following a myocardial infarction and a drop in blood pressure, she lapsed into an apparently irreversible stupor. Ms. G has no advance directives, and, according to her family and her primary care team, had never discussed her treatment preferences. To maintain Ms. G, a nasogastric tube is inserted for feeding. Over a period of time, Ms. G has several bouts of aspiration pneumonia, accompanied by shaking chills, shortness of breath, and chest congestion. The pneumonia responded only to triple antibiotics, the administration of which required repeated insertions of the IV, as well as monitoring of blood tests.

After the second episode of pneumonia, the staff questioned the use of such aggressive and invasive treatment on a patient who would most likely never regain consciousness. They felt that Ms. G's pneumonia symptoms clearly responded to the antibiotics, but they questioned the attendant discomfort of the treatment and the fact that it would enable her to live to experience another episode of pneumonia. They were reluctant, however, to let her suffer through another bout of pneumonia without treatment because it appeared that the antibiotics did relieve her symptoms.

## QUESTIONS FOR DISCUSSION

1. Do you think it is appropriate from a medical standpoint to continue to treat Ms. G with antibiotics?
2. Do you think it is appropriate from an ethical standpoint to continue to treat Ms. G with antibiotics?
3. Are there guidelines within the law that make it necessary to treat this patient?

## ANSWERS

In deciding what is medically appropriate therapy, several questions must be asked: First, what are the goals of therapy, and what is the likelihood of achieving those goals? Second, what are the burdens of the treatment(s), and are the potential benefits worth the burdens? Third, are the treatment goals consistent with the patient's wishes? When the wishes of the patient are unknown, as in this case, clinicians try to rely on an evaluation of the first two factors in determining the best course of action.

Antibiotics in general are not considered aggressive treatment. In most situations, they can be administered with minimal discomfort and, as in this case, can be very effective in relieving the uncomfortable symptoms of infection, such as fever and chest congestion. In the case of pneumonia, however, they might also be life-prolonging, and that fact must be considered. Would the patient want life prolonged under the circumstances at hand? If this is unknown, what are the benefits and burdens of continued life support to the patient?

Many clinicians might initiate a discussion of futility in this case. The staff, in essence, has already done this. Should treatment of pneumonia be considered futile if it serves only to prolong a physiological existence of total dependency and no social interaction?

Clinicians generally accept the fact that futile therapies should not be applied in the practice of medicine. However, except for the narrow concept of physiologic futility (i.e., a treatment will never be effective [Truog, Brett, & Frader, 1992]), they do not agree on what constitutes futile treatment. Schneiderman, Jecker, and Jonsen (1990) propose a rule that a treatment is futile if it does not prove effective in the last 100 applications and only serves to prolong a severely dependent state. Albert Jonsen and his colleagues (Jonsen, Siegler, & Winslade, 1986) suggest that there may be a level of existence below which all would agree treatments could be considered futile, as no one would want to persist in that state. Neither of these approaches, however, has been widely accepted. For example, Missouri and New York still require "clear and convincing" evidence of a person's wishes before treatments can be withheld, even from patients in a persistent vegetative state (PVS) (*Cruzan v. Director*, 1990; *In re O'Connor*, 1988). Court decisions to date also support the provision of treatments that health care providers have considered futile if that request is made by the patient or surrogate. In other words, physicians or institutions have not been empowered by judicial action to override a patient's or family's desire for treatment (Truog et al., 1992).

Many feel that the component of futility that is dependent on patient and societal values regarding continued life and quality of life will continue to confound a widely accepted definition of futility. Despite a growing consensus that patients in PVS should not receive aggressive medical treatment (Angell, 1991), we are most likely left with the situation that, without knowledge of Ms. G's wishes for treatment and feelings regarding quality of life, we are obliged to provide medical as opposed to purely comfort care as long as the medical care results in some benefit to the patient that may outweigh the burdens of treatment. Further debate among both the medical and lay communities is needed before generally accepted consensus is reached regarding medical treatment in such cases (Callahan, 1991; Fox & Stocking, 1993; Truog et al., 1992).

## REFERENCES

Angell, M. (1991). The case of Helga Wanglie: A new kind of "right-to-die" case. *New England Journal of Medicine, 325*, 511–515.

Callahan, D. (1991, July–August). Medical futility, medical necessity: The problem without a name. *Hastings Center Report*, pp. 30–35.

*Cruzan v. Director*, Missouri Department of Health, 110 S. Ct. 2841, 2855–56 (1990).

Fox, E., & Stocking, C. (1993). Ethics consultants' recommendations for life-prolonging treatment of patients in a persistent vegetative state. *Journal of the American Medical Association, 270* (21), 2578–2582.

*In re O'Connor*, 72 N.Y.2d 517, 531 N.E.2d 607, 534 N.Y.S.2d (1988).

Jonsen, A. R., Siegler, M., & Winslade, W. J. (1986). *Clinical ethics.* New York: Macmillan.

Schneiderman, L. J., Jecker, N. S., & Jonsen, A. R. (1990). Medical futility: Its meaning and ethical implications. *Annals of Internal Medicine, 1112*, 949–954.

Truog, R. D., Brett, A. S., & Frader, J. (1992). The problem with futility. *New England Journal of Medicine, 326*(23), 1560–1564.

# 8

# Treating People with Dementia: When Is It Okay to Stop?

*Daniel Callahan*

Some subjects in ethics elicit a far greater degree of emotional discomfort than others. It is not the delicacy or complexity of the subject as such that seems to be the problem. There are many such problems around. It is, instead, a tacit recognition that, try as we might, it is especially hard to disentangle our personal response from the issues themselves, and that makes it especially hard to avoid self-deception and self-interest in our analysis of them.

Terminating treatment for the demented is such an issue. Dementia is universally feared, more so than almost any other disease. Few of us can tolerate the thought that we might become its victim. Even if we can bring love and devotion to the care of the demented, they also bring us fear that we might someday be ourselves so afflicted, and (usually despite ourselves) they can incite a sense of loathing and horror. It is particularly difficult in that context to separate our own feeling about the condition and what is, in distinction, the actual good of the patient. The harder it is for us to imagine finding life for ourselves tolerable in such circumstances, the harder it will be to determine what is beneficial for the patient. This concern will hover in the background of my analysis, only barely below the surface.

My focus here will be to develop some criteria for terminating life-sustaining treatment of the demented. The general question is this: under what circumstances should life-sustaining treatment for the demented be ended and the patient allowed to die? The more specific, troubling question is: Ought the fact of dementia make a difference in our decision? To answer these questions, a context is needed to fill out the full dimensions of the issue. In the first part of this chapter, I sketch a picture of a background context to help us situate the care of the demented and the termination of their treatment. In the second part, I develop some criteria to make termination decisions.

## A CONTEXT FOR ANALYSIS

I want to suggest that the pertinent context here is threefold: (1) our knowledge of the inner life and selfhood of those suffering from dementia; (2) the messages, symbolic and literal, about dementia that could be given to society by alternative kinds of policies and practices; and (3) the pertinence of economic considerations in making decisions about the good of individual patients.

### Dementia and the Self

There are two major problems to be noted here. The first, to which I will not devote much attention, bears on the place and force of advance directives in the care of the demented. Ideally, people should draw up advance directives, either a living will or the appointment of a surrogate to act in their behalf should they become incompetent. Those advance directives should stipulate what one wants to be done in the case of dementia (and I will take it for granted here that most, if not all, people are not likely to want aggressive lifesaving or life-extending treatment with advanced dementia).

Yet there is a potential puzzle here, nicely brought out in the writings of Ronald Dworkin and Sanford H. Kadish, both distinguished legal scholars. The issue, too briefly summarized here, is whether, when the time comes to make a termination decision, it is the patient's earlier advance directive that should be the determining consideration or the patient's presently expressed or implied desires. That would not likely be a dilemma if the patient cannot express desires at all but would be if the patient stated a desire to continue living or if, from all of the behavioral evidence, the patient was satisfied enough with his or her present condition and seemed on the face of it to have no urge to be dead.

Dworkin (1993) distinguishes between a patient's "experiential" interests—the patient's present state of experienced pleasure, pain, or satisfaction—and the patient's "critical" interests, those interests expressive of a patient's long-standing, settled convictions about what he or she values in life. An advance directive signed while a patient was in good health and reflecting some carefully thought-out personal values could come in conflict with the actual condition and inclinations of a patient at the critical moment. If I have stated, while in good health and after careful reflection, that I would not care to have my life extended if I become demented, should that declaration be respected even if, when the time comes, I seem to be happy enough in my demented state? Dworkin takes the position that the critical interests should be determinative and the advance directive respected; Kadish (1992) takes the other side.

Kadish, I believe, has the better of the argument, primarily for reasons bearing on the selfhood of the demented person, a self that he presumes continues to exist and that I will comment on below. A secondary reason is that a key feature in the development of the idea of advance directives has been to stress the possibility of changing or revoking those directives at any time while capacitated, not to assume that they are to function in a fixed, unchangeable way, come what may. That same reasoning could be extended to include behavior of the incapacitated that would imply either a change of mind or an implicit unwillingness to see the original criteria of the advance directives invoked in actuality. But I will not explore the problem of advance directives any further here other than to note that how we analyze the problem will, in great part, turn on our interpretation of the selfhood of the demented patients and what various states of that selfhood might morally entail.

I will instead focus my analysis on what should be done when we have no prior knowledge of a person's wishes about termination or even about the person's values. I am thus taking on the hardest of all cases, where it is left entirely to us to decide what to do based on our own values or, more precisely, on those values we conscientiously believe should apply here. That focus also helps to bring into sharp relief how we might best think about dementia and termination. The tendency in much of the discussion of termination is to focus on patient wishes, known or inferred. Obviously, that is important, but in the long run, what patients and would-be patients decide is in their best interests, or their ideas of the kind of life best worth living, will be a function of how, more generally, we come to think of a life weighted down with dementia. What *ought* I to want when I am dying of dementia? That question will hover just below the surface. We cannot achieve a perfect dissociation of our judgment about ourselves and our judgment about other people, and it would be insensitive to accept a perfect bifurcation.

I begin with my first background question: How are we best to understand the selfhood of the demented person and understand it at different stages in the development of dementia? In what sense can it be said that the demented person has a self? I will here define full selfhood as the capacity to have feelings and to be aware of them, to reason and to be able to make decisions, and to enter into relationships with other persons. A person who has even one of those capacities can be said to have a self, even if limited and impaired.

The moral corollary of this definition of selfhood is that, unlike the permanently unconscious person in a persistent vegetative state (PVS), a person with even a minimal self should be assumed to have the same desire to live as those of us more fortunate to have a full self; there should be, that is, the same presumption in favor of treatment as would be the case with anyone else. I stress *presumption* here to indicate that there can be reasons to overturn that presumption, including inferred evidence from the emotional or other expressions of the patient himself or herself, a point to which I will return later.

What can be said of the selfhood of those suffering dementia? The reality may be more complex, less wholly destructive than is often believed. Joseph Foley (1992) strikes a note of caution in this respect. "We too often assume," he writes, "that the absence of emotional display means that no emotion is being experienced. We too often assume that because communication is absent, internal mental process has stopped" (p. 37). Foley does not claim we know what is going on inside the demented person. He stresses instead two important points. The first is the lack of good research on the insight of the demented person into his or her condition, a striking deficit in our knowledge compared with the emphasis on understanding insight found, for instance, in psychiatry or psychology more generally. The second is the importance of recognizing the variability, from patient to patient and time to time, in the dementia of the individual person. No less significant, "it is important to identify functions that are lost, but even more so to identify functions that are preserved" (Foley, p. 42).

Tom Kitwood and Kathleen Bredin (1992), of the Bradford Dementia Group at Bradford University in England, strike an even more optimistic note. They emphasize three points: (1) that there can be a considerable reversal of even the severely deteriorated when their social relationships and conditions of life are changed, (2) that the condition can be stabilized in those given an intensive program of activities (40 hours or so a week), and (3) that some animal studies show the significant positive effect of companionship and activity and an improved environment. They conclude that "evidence from the care context, then, is beginning to suggest that a dementing illness is not necessarily a process of inevitable and global deterioration" (p. 280). In still another study, Steven R. Sabat and Rom Harre (1992) provide evidence to show that the self of personal identity "persists far into the end stage of the disease." The self, they contend, can be lost "but only indirectly as a result of the disease. The primary cause of the loss of self is the ways in which others view and treat the Alzheimer's sufferer" (p. 443).

I make no claim here that the kinds of evidence cited in these articles are definitive, nor do the authors. But it is surely sufficient to suggest that, for ethical purposes, the sufferer of dementia cannot decisively be declared either out of touch with the self or definitively out of the human community (especially because communication with dementia patients remains possible almost to the very end, however rudimentary). As outside observers, of course, we may be appalled by the kind of self we observe, indeed often fearful but this is *our* reaction, not necessarily that of the demented person to himself or herself. A distinction must, of course, be made between the earlier and later stages of the condition, and it is surely possible that, by the last stages, the deterioration is so far advanced that the familiar stereotype is realized:

that of a person whose deterioration has destroyed both body and self. Even then we may not know exactly when the self was irretrievably lost, when some significant borderline was crossed.

I draw from this analysis one simple conclusion: There is no self-evident reason that, based on the selfhood of the dementia victim, he or she should be treated in any significantly different way from any other incompetent patient, unless and until the indirect evidence allows us to reasonably surmise that the demented patient is *consciously* suffering as a consequence of prolonged life. This would be a way of respecting the remaining selfhood. The demented person should also clearly be distinguished from the PVS patient, where the evidence of comparable personhood, direct or inferred, does not exist.

This conclusion presupposes a partial answer to a question posed at the outset, whether the fact of dementia, as distinguished from other medical conditions, should make a difference in our termination decisions. If the most important issue is the selfhood of a patient, then dementia poses problems no different in kind from those posed by other medical conditions or situations where the disease is degenerative, the future bleak, and the patient incompetent. We can well understand the special fear that we all have about becoming demented and the profound assault of dementia upon the integrity of the self. Yet I find it hard to single out a feature of dementia that makes it singularly different from other diseases that can bring about a destruction of the mind and then the body so that some special standards are needed. At the same time, it should be noted, there is something about the constellation of symptoms and losses that seems to make the whole of the illness greater than the sum of its parts; therein may lie its special horror. But it is not easy to specify a way of working with that insight to develop appropriate termination standards.

### Dementia: Public Meaning and Public Symbols

In the case of the dementias, we face an old public dilemma. There is an ancient saying to the effect that we should love the sinner but not the sin. Paraphrased for my purposes, our public dilemma is this: how are we to hate and work against dementia while not, at the same time, coming to slight or demean those who suffer from it or to create excessive anxiety on the part of those who might one day come down with it? Already, a fear of dementia seems to be a potent force behind the desire of many to have legal euthanasia and physician-assisted suicide available. A death in the throes of Alzheimer's disease is seen as the mark of a death without dignity—first the self destroyed and then the body, leaving only a wreck of a person to go to his death.

The policies we come to adopt about the termination of treatment of the demented will come to play both a literal role in the way we care for them and also a symbolic role in indicating how we, as a society, have come to situate and value them. There are three possibilities in the symbolism that could develop.

First, if we come to make it much easier to terminate treatment of the demented than for other classes of incompetent patients, we will be underscoring our social loathing of the condition and our consequent devaluing of a life burdened with that condition. We will also, on the other side of the ledger, be signaling our desire to reduce the anxiety of those in the earlier stages of the condition, as well as that of family members, about their last days (or months); we will be saying that *this* condition deserves special relief. The dilemma here is that the price of reducing the anxiety about contracting the condition and promising easier release is to stigmatize the condition all the more and thus possibly, very possibly, making it more difficult to engender the attitudes of social acceptance necessary to make the life of the demented (and their families, who will share any stigmatization) more tolerable.

Second, if we treat dementia just like other conditions—giving the benefit of any doubt to the continuation of standard medical treatment—then we will inevitably provoke a continuing (and possibly escalating) terror as the number of demented people increases with the rise in the number and proportion of the elderly; more and more of us will see ourselves at risk, particularly if we have been healthy enough to stay alive into our 80s. The source of the terror will be obvious enough: there will be no ready or quick release from the dementia, and the body will be treated as if the self of which it is a part is to be preserved at all costs.

To follow the latter course would be to accept the notion that there remains a self almost to the end—and how could we not treat that self, even though diminished, much like other selves? The dilemma here is clear enough: the price of recognizing an ongoing self may be to (a) undergird the usual forces of technological medicine, which work with the simple rule "when in doubt, treat," while (b) at the same time enhancing the fear of the condition by seeming to close off a fast release from it.

Third, we could develop some kind of compromise position, aiming to minimize further stigmatization of dementia while simultaneously reducing the widespread fear that the life of the demented will be unconscionably prolonged. That will not be easy to do, but I will propose an approach below that may strengthen the possibilities in that direction.

## Economics: Priorities and Standards

There can be little doubt that the United States, like all other developed countries, faces increasingly heavy economic pressures on its health care system. The growing number of elderly, particularly those over 80, and the growing number of the demented as a direct result of that demographic change must force some unpleasant choices about the future care of the demented. Increasingly, it is possible to hear people say that, given a shortage of resources, it makes no sense to invest in extended care for the demented, a burden upon themselves, their families, and society. Alternatively, some would no doubt say that the demented should be treated like all other patients and that, in any case, no price can be put on a human life, damaged or not. If the former view is too crude and insensitive, the latter is increasingly unrealistic and potentially unjust to other sick people, who might be deprived of needed resources by an imbalance of care given to the demented. How can we try to think about this problem?

I do not believe it possible or reasonable any longer to consider the economic dimensions of medical conditions and diseases one at a time, in isolation from each other. To ask, that is, how much money we should spend to care for the demented apart from all other medical conditions of other patients who require care will get us nowhere, any more than we can say how much should be spent on cancer apart from any other disease. A health care system must respond to the aggregate ensemble of conditions, and it must do so by putting them next to each other so that their claims can be seen in a comparative way. The economists are right with their concept of an "opportunity cost," that is, the need to consider how any amount of money spent on one medical condition might more usefully or fairly, or both, have been spent on some other medical condition.

The hard problem is to find a way to implement that insight, in our case trying to decide what counts as a reasonable expenditure on the demented in comparison with spending comparable funds on other patients. Here again we encounter another problem about assigning a unique status to dementia. Is it so uniquely oppressive and fearful that we should *therefore* spend more money on those in its last stages than on other fatal conditions? Or is its downward course so inevitable and so destructive that we should *therefore* spend less money on it, spending our money where it could do more good? Given the impact on families, I would be inclined toward the former course, but I cannot find anything in dementia as such that would support that bias—though the burden on the family, an extrinsic but hardly irrelevant consideration, provides a nudge in that direction.

A priority-setting approach, of the kind used in the state of Oregon with its Medicaid program, appears the most feasible way of managing this problem. How can we rank the different medical conditions, physical and psychological, that afflict people? Which are comparatively more or less important? Such a ranking would encompass public opinion, some form of cost-benefit analysis, the likelihood of efficacious treatment, the degree of pain and suffering a condition incurs, and the like. This is not the place to develop a full theory of priority setting. My own guess is that public opinion would give a high priority to providing decent nursing and palliative care for the demented but a much lower priority to the use of high-technology medicine to prolong the life of the demented.

I would argue, in any case, that the expenditure of large amounts of money to deliberately prolong the life of the late-stage demented person would not pass an opportunity cost test or qualify as a high-priority matter. The inevitable downhill course of the disease would be one reason—death could not be averted, only delayed—and neither cure of the dementia nor amelioration of its effect could be achieved by deliberate prolongation efforts. The increasingly diminished selfhood of the patient would be another reason: the more diminished the self, as part of a trajectory of gradual diminishment, the less likely that prolongation would be able even to significantly maintain, much less restore, the selfhood that has been lost. I conclude that society would, under any comparative analysis, most likely conclude that, faced with resource scarcity, life-extending care for the demented could not compete well in the face of other medical needs in society. Nor should it.

## DEVISING CRITERIA FOR TREATMENT TERMINATION

In proposing three contextual and background considerations, I have tried to elaborate on those dimensions of dementia that should most concern us in thinking about termination. The welfare of the demented person must, however, take precedence over the others (though not wholly to override them), and thus the question of selfhood is central. But because economic forces will impinge on treatment decisions and because any policy affecting the demented will telegraph social meanings and symbols, they cannot be left out of our considerations.

I want now to focus on individual treatment decisions, indicating where the economic and social dimensions might make a difference in the analysis. In my analysis I will assume that there are differences among individuals in their response to dementia and that any criteria must have sufficient flexibility to take that into account. I will also assume that the degree to which the disease has advanced will be an important variable; late-stage dementia is not the same as early-stage dementia, and that difference counts. I will assume, finally, that whoever is making the termination decision will have done everything possible to take into account the bias of his or her own emotional responses to the patient's condition, recognizing that it is the good of the patient, not that of the decision maker, that matters.

Just because of the problem of bias, it would be unwise to make use of the notion of "quality of life" commonly used in this kind of concept. Because we do not have good insight into the mind of the demented person, we cannot assume a priori that dementia is inevitably and necessarily *perceived* by the person himself as a poor quality of life. That may be the case early on with the condition but, ironically, perhaps less so when the disease is far advanced and the patient is perhaps less aware of his or her deterioration. As mentioned above, our lack of insight into the consciousness of the demented person should make us hesitate about quality-of-life judgments. Here, in particular, there is also the temptation to mistake our own distress and recoil from the patient's condition for that of the patient, who may or may not feel the same, and we have no definitive way of knowing the truth.

Three standards can be proposed for making termination decisions: (1) no one should, in the modern world, have to live longer in the advanced stages of dementia than he or she would have in a pretechnological era; (2) the more advanced the damage of the dementia, the more legitimate it is to overturn the usual bias in favor of treatment; (3) whoever is making the decision has as strong an obligation to attempt to avoid a painful and degrading death as to promote a respect for the value of life.

*No one should, in the modern world, have to live longer in the advanced stages of dementia than he or she would have in a pretechnological era.* Every person suffering from dementia should be given adequate care, comfort, and palliation. That standard should never be changed and always be honored. It has been an enduring standard of medical practice for 2,500 years in the West and is particularly pertinent here, given the chronic, degenerative nature of the condition (Callahan, 1990). But what about the use of those medical skills and technologies that are the mark of modern medicine and that are ordinarily used to cure disease and to extend life? Are they equally required? They range from the inexpensive, painless use of antibiotics to the more elaborate and expensive techniques of open-heart surgery, dialysis, and organ transplantation.

My contention will be that there can be no obligation, in the later stages of the dementias, to prolong with technology—even simple, nonburdensome technologies—the life of someone whose course is most likely going to be steadily downhill, steadily worse. If at all possible, a patient should be spared that likelihood, and thus opportunistic infections, organ failures, and other life-threatening conditions should not be opposed with technology, whose use should be restricted to palliation. It is hard to imagine how the use of modern technologies that extend life could be more beneficial for the advanced-stage patient—greatly enhancing the likelihood of an even worse outcome—than their omission. Modern medicine should be an option for severely deteriorated patients only if it promises clear benefit; it should not be an imposed burden (Callahan, 1993). The costs of high-technology terminal care are not a trivial consideration. Such costs can be justified only if some clear benefit is to result, and there seems to be none here.

*The likely deterioration should lead to a shift in the usual standard of treatment, that of stopping rather than continuing treatment.* The ordinary standard of treatment with an incompetent patient is, lacking specific instructions otherwise, to treat rather than not to treat, with the burden of proof on those who would want to stop the treatment. With advanced dementia that burden should be reversed that is, the presumption should be against treatment unless there are some compelling reasons to continue the treatment. The traditional reasoning behind the older and ordinary rule is that most people prefer to go on living rather than to die; thus, it is a not-surprising standard. In this case, in which the effect of continuing treatment would be to prolong the life of the patient and thus at the same time prolong the deterioration of the patient, there can be no obvious benefits; the treatment paves the way for further deterioration, not improvement or even stability.

*There is as great an obligation to avoid a lingering, painful, or degrading death as there is to promote health and life.* Among the important goals of medicine are those of preserving life, sustaining health, and relieving pain and suffering. I propose one other goal: the duty to seek, within moral means, a decent, peaceful death, an aspect of the duty to try to relieve suffering. A death that is lingering, painful, or psychologically degrading is not a good death; and if medicine fails to do what it can within moral limits to avoid such a death, it has failed in an important part of its mission. This means avoiding a technological obsessiveness that would seek to maintain the body and its organs well past the point of any benefit. It also means promoting an effort to gauge the effect of continuing treatment on the quality of the death it might make possible or likely.

In thinking about the likely downhill course of the disease, ought the diminished self of the patient make a difference? I am ambivalent on this point. I argued above that, because the demented person has a residual, though severely impaired self, he or she should be treated like any other impaired person, and treatment should be continued. But there is a side of me—and of most others, I would surmise—that wants to say that the degree of impairment of the self should somehow, somewhere make a difference in our reckoning. This impulse no doubt springs from a common reaction to the deteriorated self of the demented person: I do not want to end *my* life like that. Though understandable as an impulse, I can find no good reason to allow it to overcome the previously stated principle that, if there is any self at all, the demented person should not be singled out for special termination criteria because of the dementia.

No physician can guarantee a peaceful death, but there are many things that can be done to increase its possibility. The most important is simply to promote a responsibility to balance off the possible benefits of continued treatment against the possibility that the treatment may worsen the process of dying. Those two possibilities should be set in fruitful tension with each other. This will require asking not simply about the immediate benefit that treatment will bring (for it might reduce a fever or thwart a spreading infection) but also about the long-term consequences of the intervention. A treatment that provides an immediate benefit only to set the patient up for a worse death in the future should not be considered a value for the patient. Nor, economically, can it be considered a desirable social value.

## APPLICATION OF THE CRITERIA

What I am looking for with these criteria is to address three major problems of termination decisions: how and when to use available technologies that could sustain the life of the patient; how and when to turn upside down the traditional standard that, when in doubt, treatment should be provided; and how to determine when to invoke the duty of the physician to help the patient avoid a poor death. At present, treatment is often initiated or sustained because of a pervasive belief that possibly effective treatment should be used, that doubt should be resolved in favor of treatment, and that the physician's primary duty lies in improving or maintaining a decent quality of life rather than in promoting a peaceful death. I do not claim that this belief exists everywhere or that the principles I am suggesting are not already, at least tacitly, often used. The existence of a hospice movement shows that there are other extant standards (even though hospice is too infrequently used by the dying demented). I only want to note what appear to be the prevailing standards and why those standards need to be significantly modified in the case of patients dying with dementia (though not uniquely with them).

There still remain some problems with the proposed criteria. The most obvious is in trying to determine when the time has come to invoke them: when is there *enough* deterioration to invoke the criteria? No precise moment can be specified; like much else in medicine, it will be a matter of judgment. But some indicators can be suggested. One of them would be the emotional state of the patient. If there is evidence that the patient is suffering, whether evinced by the ordinary sounds of suffering (moaning, for instance) or by the body language of discomfort and agitated restlessness, then that apparent suffering should be taken seriously. If the demented continue to have some kind of a self, they should be accorded all of the usual deference given to those who, apparently suffering, cannot verbally express themselves. Thus, evidence of suffering, verbal or nonverbal, should be a significant signal to terminate (or not to initiate) life-sustaining treatment.

Another indicator would be the degree of probability, based on clinical experience, that further treatment will enhance the likelihood of a poor death rather than an improved quality of life. Because this is a matter of probabilities, it will often not be easy to calculate. But because the general course of the dementias is downhill, there should be—keeping that point in mind—as much care to avoid increasing the odds of a poor death as care to not terminate treatment too quickly. Thus, the standard for when the time has come to terminate treatment should not be set so high that the risk of a poor death is increased.

I have sought to find a middle way, a compromise position, between the hazard of treating the demented too aggressively, as if their dementia counted for nothing in our judgment, and failing to give them sufficient treatment on the grounds that their dementia puts them out of the human community. The suggested standards for terminating treatment are meant to reassure those suffering from dementia in its early stages that we will not medically sustain their lives only to allow them a worse death or that we will, in our horror of dementia, allow that emotion to lead us to ignore or deny the self that may remain, even if damaged and all but hidden from our sight. I have looked for a stance that signals to demented persons or their families that we can and will terminate treatment if at all possible before total deterioration has taken place, but that we will not do so in a way that suggests we have a special horror of the condition, creating criteria that allow us to stop treatment well before what would be seen as acceptable with other patients.

Two unpleasant questions might be asked at this point. Is it possible to imagine a time when insurance or government reimbursement might not be made available for medical efforts to sustain the life of those with advanced cases of dementia? Yes, it is possible, particularly if a priority-setting approach was taken and life-sustaining treatment for the demented came low on the list of covered services, a likely result. The second question is whether a general approach to termination of treatment for the demented that shifted the benefit of doubt toward nontreatment would stigmatize the demented, suggesting that they need to be rushed out of life, so horrible is such an existence? That is a hazard, but if that approach was balanced by one that attended carefully to the selfhood of the demented, sensitive to what remained instead of what was lost (as Joseph Foley [1992] suggests), the chances of stigmatization could be minimized.

## REFERENCES

Callahan, D. (1990). *What kind of life: The limits of medical progress.* New York: Simon and Schuster.

Callahan, D. (1993). *The troubled dream of life: Living with mortality.* New York: Simon and Schuster.

Dworkin, R. (1993). *Life's dominion: An argument about abortion, euthanasia, and individual freedom.* New York: Alfred A. Knopf.

Foley, J. M. (1992). The experience of being demented. In R. H. Binstock, S. G. Post, & P. J. Whitehouse (Eds.), *Dementia and aging: Ethics, values, and policy choices.* Baltimore: Johns Hopkins University Press.

Kadish, S. H. (1992). Letting patients die: Legal and moral reflections. *California Law Review, 80,* 857–888.

Kitwood, T., & Bredin, K. (1992). Toward a theory of dementia care: Personhood and well-being. *Aging and Society, 12,* 269–287.

Sabat, S. R., & Harre, R. (1992). The construction and deconstruction of self in Alzheimer's disease. *Aging and Society, 12,* 443–461.

## THE CASE OF MR. H

Mr. H is a 90-year-old man with dementia who has been a resident in your nursing home for almost 6 years. In that time, he never recognized any family members, nor has he been able to communicate with the staff. He is ambulatory, at times incontinent of urine, and unable to dress and feed himself. He entered your facility without any advance directives.

Mr. H's only relative is a sister who lives out of state. She has not visited Mr. H in 2 years, and all of her dealings with your nursing home have been via telephone or letter.

For most of the time that Mr. H has resided in your facility, his condition has been fairly stable. However, in the past year or so, he has had several bouts of pneumonia that were successfully treated with antibiotics, usually in the nursing home but sometimes at the hospital. In addition, he was hospitalized once for a broken hip.

His doctor calls Mr. H's sister to inform her that he is again suffering from pneumonia and will be treated with antibiotics at the hospital. When she hears this, Mr. H's sister asks the doctor to stop all treatment. She states emphatically that there is no point in prolonging her brother's life, which she describes as a "meaningless, painful existence." Further, she says, this continued treatment is extremely costly and, in her opinion, a waste of money. She says that, by prolonging her brother's life, you are using resources and spending health care dollars that could be put to much better use elsewhere.

## QUESTIONS FOR DISCUSSION

1. Do you think that Mr. H's sister has a valid concern?
2. Would you take into consideration the reasons cited by Mr. H's sister to stop treatment?
3. What would you do in this case?
4. Would knowing more of Mr. H's social history be helpful?

## ANSWERS

Mr. H's sister has valid concerns. However, her concerns raise other issues. The first of these involves rationing. Though most authorities in medical ethics as well as government accept that the need to ration health care is inevitable, it is also well recognized that the rationing should not take place at the bedside. It is not the role of the family or clinician to make this decision unless it fulfills the previously expressed wish of the patient. Mr. H's sister's views regarding Mr. H's quality of life raise similar concerns. Though there may be some generally accepted level of existence that everyone would agree is an unacceptable quality of life, what constitutes an acceptable quality of life should be determined by the patient (Jonsen, Siegler, & Winslade, 1986). Again, it is not the role of family or health care providers to make this judgment, absent information from the patient himself or herself.

It might also be helpful to learn more about Mr. H's social history to get a sense of what his life was like and what was important to him. Optimally, it would be helpful if it were possible to get a values history from any people who might have known Mr. H. A values history can give a sense of how Mr. H would want to be treated at a point when he could not make decisions for himself even though he may never have discussed particular treatments (Gibson, 1990). For example, people who knew him when he was cognitively intact might know whether quality of life was more important to him than quantity of life. If, however, there is no one who can really paint an accurate picture of Mr. H's values and there is no evidence of his wishes, the most appropriate option in this case is to continue to provide treatment to him as long as it does not violate accepted standards for medical care, and that the treatments are not burdensome.

## REFERENCES

Gibson, J. M. (1990). National values history project. *Generations, 14*(Suppl.), 51–64.

Jonsen, A. R., Siegler, M., & Winslade, W. J. (1986). *Clinical ethics.* New York: Macmillan.

# 9

# Treating People with Dementia: Can We Afford Not to Stop?

*Marianne C. Fahs*

As we approach a new era of health care reform strategies, there remains confusion over what the nature of our goals should be for this uniquely American health care system (Leaf, 1993). The major agenda put forward for public debate to date by the Clinton administration concerns the demarcation of a new organizational structure of government regulations balanced with competitive market incentives. The administration's proposed mix of private and public structures has the dual objectives of controlling costs and assuring quality. The reorganization is, of course, subject to the constraints of political feasibility. Realistic strategies for achieving the intended objectives of the reorganization will require a new consensus on the respective roles prevention and treatment will play in the new health care system (Angell, 1993; Fries et al., 1993; Leaf, 1993).

A serious reappraisal is needed of the short- and long-term opportunities for prevention and treatment in the decades that lie ahead—the decades of the "elderly boom." The aging of the U.S. population is a significant demographic force that will have a serious and wide-ranging impact on health care needs and use in the years ahead. It remains to us to reexamine our health goals and national budget allocations if we are to avoid intolerably high rates of disability and soaring health care costs in the future

(Schneider & Guralnik, 1990; Zedlewski, Barnes, Burt, McBride, & Meyer, 1993). As health care reform evolves, it is of particular importance that we critically examine the nation's comparative budget allocation between short-term acute treatment costs and long-term investments in the prevention or postponement of disability (Fahs, 1992).

The circumstances we confront with respect to the tragedy of Alzheimer's disease provide a prototypical example of such allocation decisions we as a nation have yet to face (USDHHS, 1991a; Weiler, 1987). The purpose of this chapter is to present an economic analysis of the policy choices before us as we grapple with this debilitating and socially draining disease. Before we can analyze properly the issue of whether we can afford not to stop treating patients with Alzheimer's disease, it is important to gain perspective and examine the broader economic implications of this disease for our society.

The organization of this chapter is as follows: The first section presents a critical review of estimates to date of the economic costs of Alzheimer's disease; the second presents projections of the cost of Alzheimer's disease in the future; the third presents a discussion of issues of equity in our health care system with respect to Alzheimer's disease; and the last section suggests future directions for health care policy.

## THE ECONOMIC COSTS OF ALZHEIMER'S DISEASE

Economic theory offers a useful theoretical approach to examining the consequences of disease in our society. This approach is called *opportunity cost* (Henderson & Quandt, 1971). Opportunity cost is simply a measure of the opportunities we as a society forgo because our resources are unavailable or tied up in other areas. As we will see in this analysis, the national opportunity costs of Alzheimer's disease are enormous.

Another important theoretical contribution of economics to understanding the consequences of the disease in our society is the concept of direct and indirect costs (Hodgson & Meiners, 1982; Rice, 1985). Direct costs are simply health care expenditures such as physician costs, laboratory costs, nursing costs, prescription costs, and so on. Indirect costs are the lost productivity to society resulting from disability or premature death. Indirect costs include the lost productivity of the ill individual and of other members of the individual's family or friends involved in patient care and support.

In 1987, Hay and Ernst published estimates in the *American Journal of Public Health* on the total cost of Alzheimer's disease to our country. Using an incidence-based approach (all first-diagnosed Alzheimer's disease patients in 1983), Hay and Ernst estimated that the disease cost our country over $31 billion in 1983. They estimated the total cost per disease per patient in 1983 dollars as between $49,000 and $493,000, depending on the age and sex of the patient in question. Males aged 45 to 50 at first diagnosis had the highest cost, and males aged greater than 85 had the lowest cost. Using an 8% medical care price index inflator, these figures are approximately double in 1993 dollars. Using the Hay and Ernst methodology, we can estimate that Alzheimer's disease now costs between $100,000 and $1 million per patient.

However, Hay and Ernst's (1987) figures are underestimates in two respects. In one respect, their incidence-based total cost projection may very likely have been too conservative. There is a controversy in the literature regarding incidence and prevalence rates for Alzheimer's disease (Backman et al., 1992; Evans et al., 1989). Hay and Ernst were compelled to calculate incidence rates using prevalence data from foreign sources because of the dearth of research on this disease in the United States. The prevalence of Alzheimer's disease for men 75 and over was estimated to be 5.8%, and for women 75 and over the prevalence estimate is 9.7%. However, more recent data indicate that the prevalence of Alzheimer's disease or related dementia among people 85 and over may be 25% to 40% (Evans et al., 1989; Rice et al., 1993).

The second source of potential bias stems from the use of secondary data sources to estimate the indirect costs associated with informal home care by family and friends. Hay and Ernst (1987) extracted secondary data from studies of home care costs for "impaired" persons with both physical and mental disabilities. Although Hay and Ernst assert that "the estimates probably measure the home care costs of Alzheimer's disease reasonably well" (p. 1172), more recent evidence indicates that these estimates are likely far too low.

Rice et al. (1993) collected primary data to estimate the cost of Alzheimer's disease, particularly the indirect costs. They found that informal caregivers, usually middle-aged daughters, spend an average of 286 hours per month caring for a noninstitutionalized elderly person with Alzheimer's disease and 36 hours per month on average for an institutionalized person with Alzheimer's disease. Using replacement costs (the cost of replacing the daughters' services with home care attendants), Rice and her colleagues estimate that indirect costs associated with Alzheimer's disease constitute fully 65% of the economic costs to our society for this disease. The estimates of Rice et al. indicate that we are currently spending approximately $100 billion per year on Alzheimer's disease, using a prevalence-based method.

The use of replacement costs to estimate the opportunity costs to the market of informal caregivers is controversial. Although market wages for women may underestimate the value of women's time because of gender disparities in income, replacement costs may also underestimate the true opportunity costs to society of losing the productivity of middle-aged daughters, a larger and larger proportion of whom are reaching their peak productivity levels in the labor market (Fahs, 1993). Despite the limits of the Rice et al. (1993) research, the study presents the best estimates to date of the direct and indirect costs of caring for Alzheimer's disease patients.

## FUTURE PROJECTIONS

There is no historical precedent for the demographic changes we will face in the 21st century. Never before have so many people lived to be so old. Already, more than 50% of the entire U.S. population reaches 75, and 25% live to age 85 (Weiler, 1987). The segment 85 years of age and older is growing fastest and is expected to increase by 100% by 2010, under assumptions of the U.S. Bureau of the Census (1989) middle series population model. From 2011 to 2050, growth in the elderly population will become even more dramatic. The population aged 85 and over is expected to grow from over 3 million today to 8 million in 2030 and to nearly double in size *again* by 2050.

Schneider and Guralnik (1990) estimate that by the year 2040, the aging of the population could increase the number of dementia patients three- to fivefold. Using the Rice et al. (1993) figures, within the next 50 years we could be facing a $300 billion to $500 billion national expenditure for Alzheimer's disease. Clearly, the impact of Alzheimer's disease on our society is a major public health concern.

Here again, these projections may be underestimates. Serious questions have been raised regarding the census projections upon which these estimates are based. Ahlberg and Vaupel (1990), now project an average life span of 94 for men and 100 for women by the year 2080. This projection, if realized, would mean that instead of 19 million people aged 85 and over in the United States in the year 2080, there would be 71 million people aged 85 and over.

On a shorter time frame, Duke University researcher Professor Ken Manton and his colleagues (1994) believe that even without any breakthroughs in the elimination of the major killer diseases, there will, as a result of improved health maintenance over their life span, be some 42 million of the oldest-old in our population by the year 2040—against the Census Bureau's (1989) middle range projection of 12 million. That again is 3½ times larger than the Census Bureau's estimate. Thus, as a measure of the magnitude of the problem, rough projections of the economic impact in the year 2040 of $300 billion to $500 billion may again be an *underestimate*!

## ISSUES OF EQUITY

The economic consequences of maintaining the status quo have dire implications for vulnerable subgroups of our population. There are disproportionate consequences for minorities and for women. The projections discussed above mask differences in rates of increase among vulnerable subgroups of our elderly. Again using the conservative middle-growth estimates put out by the U.S. Bureau of the Census (1989), we expect a 200% increase in mortality from Alzheimer's disease and related dementias in the next 50 years. This compares to a projected 85% increase in breast cancer mortality and a 104% increase in lung cancer mortality. However, the estimate of a 200% increase in mortality from the dementias underestimates the differential impact this disease will have among minority groups in our society. For minorities, mortality from the dementias will increase by 436% as U.S. minority populations age.

In addition, women's greater longevity and the consequent disproportionate representation of women among the elderly portend greater burdens of disability due to Alzheimer's disease among elderly women. The economic and social consequences will be greater for women of all ages, both for those groups of women directly affected by the disease and for their informal caretakers, who are most often daughters. Thus, women represent a disproportionate share of the direct and indirect costs of this disease to our society (Fahs, 1993).

There are some who question what will happen if the hidden economic subsidy currently provided by the free or poorly paid caregiving services of women is withdrawn. The fact is that much of the present system of care for the elderly is financially viable today only because it depends on the exploitation of women. These are women of all ages who either give unpaid care at home or who are inadequately paid employees of nursing homes or home care agencies. Many families cannot afford home care services. Only 25% of disabled elderly receive any paid care. Because of home care responsibilities, many women are forced to leave their paid employment or take part-time jobs. This, of course, limits their income. It can also make them ineligible for private and, in some cases, state pensions. This social burden can make it impossible for women to save and thus contributes to female poverty in old age (Muller, 1990).

## HEALTH POLICY CONSIDERATIONS

In spite of these statistics, public policy has been slow to respond. Alan Pifer (1993), former president of the Carnegie Foundation, predicts the likelihood of three kinds of crisis ahead: a crisis in the availability of appropriate facilities to house the disabled elderly, a crisis in the availability of caregivers, and a cost crisis. Our federal government is now spending an average of $12,000 per elderly person per year, which adds up to about 30% of annual federal spending for all purposes. The question now is how high those figures can go before we begin to short-change investment in young people and in economic growth and thereby jeopardize our futures, including our future ability to do anything at all for the elderly.

These circumstances have led some to call for rationing. It is clear that without advances in both the basic sciences and the health services sciences, further rationing will have to occur. However, others have suggested it is too soon to ration. Rationing at this time would be inequitable, particularly for women, and would perpetuate broad gender inequities in the society (Jecker, 1991). It is my contention that it is wrong to impose social constraints on individual choices, with the goal of reducing expenditures, when the system itself has not faced these difficult choices. In other words, balancing the responsibility for an inefficient system on the backs of individual patients is unethical.

Furthermore, studies suggest that we already ration informally (Lubitz & Riley, 1993). Evidence shows that many fewer resources are used on persons with low functional status in their last year of life, compared to persons with high functional status in their last year of life (Scitovsky, 1988). Rejecting formal rationing at this juncture in our social development can be a clear beacon for improving the social policies affecting all of us.

It is too soon to ration Alzheimer's disease care. First, we must address the inefficiencies within the medical care system. Clearly, inefficiencies exist. Brooke et al. (1990) have found that close to 40% of procedures performed during hospitalization are inappropriate according to current standard practice guidelines. In addition, work done by Wennberg and Gittlesohn (1973) and Chassin et al. (1987), showing wide geographic differences in practice patterns, reveals possibilities for increased efficiency in the supply of medical care. Finally, estimates show that our current health insurance system of over 1,500 different insurance companies wastes up to $100 billion a year in administrative costs. The Clinton health care reform package is intended to limit these inefficiencies. However, because the Clinton plan preserves a multi-payer system, it is not clear that administrative inefficiency will be minimized. In fact, some foresee an increase in administrative overhead as insurers become increasingly involved at the micro-level in managing physician practice.

In fact, there is a fourth inefficiency—the underinvestment in research in this country. Currently, the total budget for research on Alzheimer's disease in the United States ranges between $150 million and $200 million. That is less than 0.2% to 0.3% of total expenditures on this disease currently. In fact, the proposed budget for the National Institutes of Health (NIH) is only $10.67 billion, which is less than 1% of health care expenditures. Although this budget represents a 3.2% increase, it may still be less than the inflation rate expected for biomedical research next year. The total budget for the National Institute of Aging (NIA) is only $399 million (1993 estimate), and in fiscal year 1994, there are projected cuts to $394 million.

This funding level has been constant over the past 5 years, with no increase, and falls far short of other allocations. For instance, for AIDS, $1.6 billion has been allocated; for cancer, $1.5 billion; and for heart disease, $610 million. We need to reorder our research priorities with respect to the public health impact of the diseases associated with aging.

We must find ways of combining cost control with patient advocacy. The need for increased public investment in health care research for age-related diseases such as Alzheimer's disease is compelling. The economic and social costs we face ahead are staggering if we do not prevent or postpone these disabilities. It must be public investment because the externalities associated with these diseases are not confined to any one market or industry but cut across broad sectors of our society. Thus, no private investment will reap the full returns; and therefore, private investment, as economic theory shows, will always be underfunded. The market for effective treatment of Alzheimer's disease has been estimated to be $8 billion annually. That falls far short of the actual annual economic cost to our society of this disease.

It is not just biological research that must be increased; it is also services research. With the exception of one large demonstration project at the Health Care Financing Agency, no federal funding for services development has occurred. As recently as fiscal year 1989, only $2 million of the $16 million authorized for Alzheimer's disease and related dementias services research had actually been appropriated. Thus, federal spending on health services research related to dementia is a small fraction of 1% of the federal payments for long-term care for those with dementia. Services research centers should be established, and these centers should have appropriate linkages with existing centers that are focused on basic and clinical biomedical Alzheimer's disease research. We need to become actively involved in developing new kinds of acceptable services and inexpensive living arrangements for the growing numbers of dependent elderly, such as assisted living communities.

## CONCLUSION

We must focus on the long-term goals of improved health and productivity in our society. And we must commit the resources now that are necessary to achieve these long-term goals. Let us not lose sight of the fact that health care expenditures are not just costs to the society; they are investments in the productivity of our nation.

## REFERENCES

Ahlberg, D. A., & Vaupel, J. W. (1990). Alternative projections of the U.S. population. *Demography, 4,* 439–452.

Angell, M. (1993). How much will health care reform cost? *New England Journal of Medicine, 328,* 1778–1779.

Bachman D. L., Wolf, P. A., Linn, R., Knoefel, J. E., Cobb, J., Belanger, A., D'Agostino, R. B., & White, L. R. (1992). Prevalence of dementia and probable senile dementia of the Alzheimer's type in the Framingham study. *Neurology, 42,* 115–119.

Brooke, R. H., Kamberg, C. J., Mayer-Oakes, A., Beers, M. H., Raube, K., & Steiner, A. (1990). Appropriateness of acute medical care for the elderly: An analysis of the literature. *Health Policy, 14,* 225–242.

Chassin, M. R., Kosecoff, J., Park, R. E., Winslow, C. M., Kahn, K. L., Chown, M. J., Hebert, L. E., Hennekens, C. H., & Taylor, J. O. (1987). Does inappropriate use explain geographic variations in the use of health care services? *Journal of the American Medical Association, 258,* 2551–2556.

Evans D. A., Funkenstein, H. H., Albert, M. S., Scherr, P. A., Cook, N. R., Chown, M. J., Hebert, L. E., Hennekens, C. H., & Taylor, J. O. (1989). Prevalence of Alzheimer's disease in a community population of older persons: Higher than previously reported. *Journal of the American Medical Association, 262,* 2551–2556.

Fahs, M. C. (1992). Public health in crisis: The economic consequences of inaction on preventive medicine. *Mount Sinai Journal of Medicine, 59,* 469–478.

Fahs, M. C. (1993). Preventive medical care: Targeting elderly women in an aging society. In A. Pifer & J. Allen (Eds.), *Women on the front lines: Meeting the challenge of an aging America*. Washington, DC: Urban Institute Press.

Fries, J. F., Koop, C. E., Beadle, C. E., Cooper, P. P., England, M. J., Greaves, R. F., Sokolov, J. J., Wright, D. & the Health Project Consortium. (1993). Reducing the need and demand for medical services. *New England Journal of Medicine, 329*, 321–325.

Hay, J. W., & Ernst, R. L. (1987). The economic cost of Alzheimer's disease. *American Journal of Public Health, 77*, 1169–1175.

Henderson, J. M., & Quandt, R. E. (1971). *Microeconomic theory*. New York: McGraw-Hill.

Hodgson T. A., & Meiners, M. R. (1982). Cost-of-illness methodology: A guide to current practices and procedures. *Health and Society, 60*, 429–462.

Hu, T., Huang L., & Cartwright, W. S. (1986). Evaluation of the costs of caring for the senile demented elderly: A pilot study. *Gerontologist, 26*, 158–163.

Huang, L., Cartwright, W. S., & Hu, T. (1988). The economic cost of senile dementia in the United States, 1985. *Public Health Reports, 103*, 3–7.

Jecker, N. S. (1991). Age-based rationing and women. *Journal of the American Medical Association, 266*, 3012–3015.

Leaf A. (1993). Preventive medicine for our ailing health care system. *Journal of the American Medical Association, 269*, 616–618.

Lenizner, H. R., Pamuk, E. R., Rhodenhiser, E. P., Rothenberg, R., & Powell-Griner, E. (1992). The quality of life in the year before death. *American Journal of Public Health, 82*, 1093–1098.

Lilienfeld, D. E., & Perl, D. P. (1992). Projected neurodegenerative disease mortality in the United States, 1990–2040. Unpublished manuscript, Mount Sinai School of Medicine, New York.

Lubitz, J. D., & Riley, G. F. (1993). Trends in Medicare payments in the last year of life. *New England Journal of Medicine, 328*, 1092–1096.

Manton, K. G., Stallard, E., & Singer, B. H. (1994). Projecting the future size and health status of the U.S. elderly population. In D. Wise (Ed.), *Studies of the economics of aging*. Chicago: National Bureau of Economic Research, University of Chicago Press.

Muller, C. (1990). *Health care and gender*. New York: Russell Sage Foundation.

Pifer, A. (1993, April). Preparing for the fourth age. Abbeyfield Society Lecture. Southport Institute for Women and Aging Project. London.

Rice, D. P., Fox, P. J., Max, W., Webber, P. A., Lindeman, D. A., Hauck, W. W., & Segura, E. (1993). The economic burden of Alzheimer's disease care. *Health Affairs, 12,* 164–176.

Rice, D. P., Hodgson, T. A., Kopstein, A. N. (1985). The economic costs of illness: A replication and update. *Health care financing review, 1* (1), 61–80.

Rivlin, A. M., & Wiener, J. M. (1988). *Caring for the disabled elderly: Who will pay?* Washington, DC: Brookings Institution.

Russell, L. B. (1993). The role of prevention in health reform. *New England Journal of Medicine, 329,* 352–354.

Schneider, E. L., & Guralnik, J. M. (1990). The aging of America: Impact on health care costs. *Journal of the American Medical Association, 263,* 2335–2340.

Scitovsky, A. A. (1988). Medical care in the last twelve months of life: The relation between age, functional status, and medical care expenditures. *Milbank Quarterly, 66,* 640–660.

U.S. Bureau of the Census. (1989). Projections of the population of the U.S. by age, sex, and race: 1988 to 2080. *Current Population Reports,* Ser. P-25, No. 451. Washington, DC: U.S. Government Printing Office.

U.S. Congress, Office of Technology Assessment. (1987). *Losing a million minds: Confronting the tragedy of Alzheimer's disease and other dementias* (Pub No. OTA-BA-323). Washington, DC: U.S. Government Printing Office.

U.S. Congress, Office of Technology Assessment. (1992). *Special care units for people with Alzheimer's and other dementias* (Pub No. OTA-H-544). Washington, DC: U.S. Government Printing Office.

U.S. Department of Health and Human Services. (1991a). *Second report of the Advisory Panel on Alzheimer's Disease 1990.* (DHHS Publication No. ADM 91-1791. Washington, DC: U.S. Government Printing Office.

U.S. Department of Health and Human Services. (1991b). *Proceedings of the 1991 Public Health Conference on Records and Statistics.* Washington, DC: U.S. Government Printing Office.

U.S. Government Accounting Office. (1991a). *Canadian health insurance: Lessons from the US* (GAO/HRD-91-90). Washington, DC: U.S. Government Printing Office.

U.S. Government Accounting Office. (1991b). *Long-term care: Projected needs of the aging baby boom generation* (GAO/HRD 91-86). Washington, DC: U.S. Government Printing Office.

Wennberg, J., & Gittleson, A. (1973). Small-area variations in health care delivery. *Science, 182,* 1102–1108.

Weiler, P. G. (1986). Risk factors associated with senile dementia of the Alzheimer's type. *American Journal of Preventive Medicine, 2,* 297–305.

Weiler, P. G. (1987). The public health impact of Alzheimer's disease. *American Journal of Public Health, 77,* 1157–1158.

Woolhandler, S., & Himmelstein, D. (1991). The deteriorating administrative efficiency of the U.S. health care system. *New England Journal of Medicine, 325,* 1253–1258.

Zedlewski, S. R., Barnes, R. O., Burt, M. R., McBride, T. D., & Meyer, J. A. (1990). The needs of the elderly in the 21st century. Washington, DC: Urban Institute Press.

## THE CASE OF MS. J

Ms. J is a 99-year-old woman admitted to your nursing home for rehabilitation after suffering a fractured hip. Although she is also in the early stages of dementia, her level of functioning is relatively high. She is still able to participate in her rehab program and usually recognizes several members of the primary care team responsible for her care. She also recognizes her family, although they visit very infrequently. On admission, her social worker discussed with her the possibility of executing a health care proxy and naming a family member or friend as agent to make treatment decisions for her should she become unable to do so for herself. However, for reasons she would not explain, she was reluctant to do so.

Shortly before she is scheduled to be discharged, Ms. J's speech becomes slurred and she develops weakness on her left side. Accordingly, she is admitted to the hospital, where her condition deteriorates dramatically. A CT scan reveals a massive CVA, and the physicians responsible for her care feel that her prognosis is extremely grim. They tell her family that she will most likely die within a short time and recommend that the most appropriate course of action, all things considered, is to keep her as comfortable as possible and "let nature take its course." Three of her grandchildren, one of whom is a physician, disagree with this recommendation. They demand that their grandmother be intubated and placed on a ventilator and that every effort be made to keep her alive, no matter what the cost.

## QUESTIONS FOR DISCUSSION

1. What should the physicians at the hospital do about Ms. J?
2. How could the nursing home staff be of assistance in this case? Should they be involved in the decision-making process?

## ANSWERS

The use of sophisticated medical technology is extremely costly, and it has been suggested that age-based rationing of scarce resources should be employed (Callahan, 1987). Some may feel that it is a flagrant waste of such technology to apply it to a 99-year-old woman. However, of issue here is less the age of the patient than the futility of maintaining anyone with such a serious prognosis on a ventilator for any length of time. The problem of determining whether care is futile in any particular situation has been addressed elsewhere (see the Case of Ms. G).

Judith Ross (1993) suggests another way to address the topic of futility, and that is to replace it with the notion of appropriateness of treatments. She states that appropriate treatments should not be associated with poor outcomes, as could likely be the situation in this case. She encourages physicians and institutions to be more proactive in developing guidelines that can not only be put forth for public debate but actually implemented via institutional missions statements. Daniel Callahan (1991) suggests that we pursue the question of futility by looking at the definition of "medical necessity," a concept he feels cannot, as with futility, be addressed by medical information alone. He too feels that the answer lies in more public debate and addresses the political, moral, and economic issues affecting health care as well as medical facts.

Current law, however, supports family requests for treatments that appear futile, again as mentioned earlier. That does not mean, however, that physicians and other health care providers should not continue to work with families to explore their reasons for wanting therapies that are considered inappropriate under the circumstances by the caregiving majority. Families must be encouraged to reflect on the patient's values and not just their own. Unresolved conflicts might be uncovered. Misperceptions of religious obligations may be involved. Discussion of such issues are often helpful in conflict resolution (Truog, Brett, & Frader, 1992).

The primary care team responsible for the care of Ms. J in the nursing home might have some valuable information regarding her care. She may, for example, have had discussions with one or more of her caregivers about issues that are important to her. And although she may not have specifically mentioned treatment preferences, she may have given an indication of her values and how she would like to live. These conversations could potentially be helpful to her physicians in the hospital and to her family members as they attempt to make treatment decisions for her. For example, if she had indicated to her nursing assistant that a certain level of independence was key to her happiness and that she would not want to live any kind of life where she could do nothing for herself, this might provide some solace to her family and encourage them not to request aggressive treatment, given her grave prognosis.

## REFERENCES

Callahan, D. (1987). *Setting limits: Medical goals in an aging society.* New York: Simon and Schuster.

Callahan, D. (1991, July–August). Medical futility, medical necessity: The problem without a name. *Hastings Center Report*, pp. 30–35.

Ross, J. (1993). Futile treatment: Where are we? *Ethical Currents, 35*, 1–3, 7.

Truog, R. D., Brett, A. S., & Frader, J. (1992). The problem with futility. *New England Journal of Medicine, 326*(23), 1560–1564.

# 10

# Some Views on Ethics and Later Life*

*Ambassador Morris B. Abram*

As a direct result of my medical history, my views on the ethical problems of medicine have shifted from time to time. In 1973, I had acute myelogenous leukemia and was a candidate for almost certain death. Nonetheless, the National Institutes of Health and other agencies spent at least $1 million to keep me alive. That expenditure did not extend the mortality rate in this country. Therefore, I contributed nothing to society unless one argues that the experiments I underwent made some contribution.

Then, last year, at the age of 73, I had open-heart surgery at Mount Sinai Medical Center in New York City, undergoing a quadruple bypass and acquiring a porcine valve. Between insurance and other sources, at least $200,000 worth of public resources were spent on me. I doubt that increased the prospect of human life in this country to any degree. In looking at these two situations, the question that immediately comes to mind centers on the appropriateness of spending more than $1 million to treat someone for a potentially incurable disease or to expend so many health care dollars on a person in his 70s. These are questions that we will increasingly come to face as government involvement in heath care grows. And clearly, the whole question of ethics—and medical ethics in particular—is very debatable.

---

*This chapter is a transcript of an oral presentation by the author.

In writing of this in the *Washington Post*, I raised a question that ethicists would say addresses the issue of utilitarianism. Do we conduct our lives and our public conduct to produce the greatest good for the greatest number? Or do we base our medical ethics upon the need of the individual and the choice of the individual and the respect for the individual life, regardless of the public health? If we do the former, $1,200,000 was not well spent. Quite frankly, however, the latter has been the tradition in medicine, and it is a tradition I hope will continue. What is of value to the individual, at least as long as it is not totally futile, ought to be the key variable that determines how individuals are treated. Nonetheless, this is debatable in various societies and certainly is something that is subject to debate based upon one's religious convictions and upon one's tradition.

Tradition and religion can play a very large role in ethical decision making, and these issues are extremely difficult to extricate. The Eskimo tradition, for example, when there was a shortage of food and of resources, was to put the older people on an iceberg and let them go out to sea. That is regarded as totally unacceptable in our society. On the other hand, some time ago, Governor Lamm of Colorado, seeing escalating health costs, posited that perhaps it is the duty of old people to die. Not surprisingly, he was criticized for this statement. But how different is Lamm's opinion from the biblical suggestion that there is a time to sow, a time to reap, a time to live, and a time to die? In any event, the great questions that are going to be presented to medical ethicists and to practitioners in the near future are going to be questions that are not only religious and traditional but also very complicated by the traditions and the necessities of government. And they have changed vastly in my lifetime.

For example, look at the role of hospitals in this century. Growing up in my hometown, I never knew a birth in a hospital. I never knew a person who died in a hospital. Home care was the norm, and those who could afford it always preferred home care and always had home care.

And what of the very serious questions of the doctor-patient relationship? Listen to what Hippocrates said of doctor-patient interactions: perform duties calmly and adroitly, concealing most things from the patient while you're attending to him. Give necessary orders with cheerfulness and sincerity. Turn his attention away from what is being done to him. Sometimes recrudesce sharply and emphatically, and sometimes comfort with solicitude and attention, revealing nothing of the patient's future or present condition.

Now, some may say that Hippocrates was an unfeeling man. I suggest he was not. In all probability, he was giving the best possible advice because actually doctors in his time knew very little. As a result, almost anything they said would have been a mistake. In reality, even in the early 20th century—statistically, not individually—people were better off not seeing a doctor.

Now, however, as we approach the 21st century, doctors know a great deal more. Therefore, there is much more information they must impart and share ethically with their patients. Unfortunately, this incredible increase in knowledge has resulted in an enormous escalation of cost. As late as 1950, only 4% of the gross national product was consumed by medical care. Today, it approaches 14%. Further, health care costs are beginning to press against other needs: housing, education, roads, national defense. Compounding this is a universal demand for universal health care. One may ask why should there be a right to universal health care when there is no right to universal housing. Well, first of all, the lack of health care creates a different kind of relationship to society. It involves pain and suffering. Much ill health is undeserved, and much ill health may involve immediate and preventable death. Lack of health care also precludes the ability to do what the Protestant work ethic celebrates: the opportunity to work. But when one says that there is a universal right to health care, then the degree to which one is ethically entitled to health care as a matter of right must be stipulated. One recommendation, made by the President's Commission, suggests that every person has a right to treatment but not to unlimited treatment.

What should be required? Obviously, emergency traumatic care, preventive care such as inoculations, alleviation of suffering, and the treatment of any individual as long as such treatment is possible and is not futile. Borderline, however, would be such issues as the public expense for *in vitro* fertilization and the care of extremely premature babies. All too frequently, sophisticated technology is applied to babies of such low weight that the possibility of producing an advance in life also produces the real probability of neurological damage. And what of the great question of treating those in whom memory and thus personhood are gone?

The mere existence of life-sustaining technology does not necessarily mandate its use.

As I see them, the public health concerns growing out of universal health care involve three issues: quality, access, and cost. Without question the United States has the finest quality of medical care at the highest level on earth. Our country is recognized as the prime source of the great advances in medical care. Access to medical care, on the other hand, is another issue, and costs are tremendous. But in repairing the problem of access, let us not forget that quality cannot be sacrificed. If it is, not only will we suffer, but the whole world, which depends on us, will suffer.

Yes, there is a time to sow, a time to reap, a time to live, and a time to die. But the question I posed in that *Washington Post* article I now repudiate. I do so because it fails to say something that is terribly important: that the question of treatment, in my judgment, should be based not on the length of time from birth but on the length of time from death.

To conclude, as I lay in Mount Sinai Hospital fully expecting death, I realized that whoever made this world did a pretty good job as a painter. Imagine an artist who paints a picture that goes on and on and on forever without a frame around it. Such a work would not be art and would not be human. So yes, there is a time to die with dignity. That time is when life's meaning is truly exhausted. But at my age now—and I'll be 75 next month—I would strongly opt for life as long as I can think and be a person.

# Afterword

*Harvey Finkelstein*

This is a time in which the entire nation is caught up in conflicting needs and desires as we face the numerous ethical issues related to health care and the elderly. On one hand, there is the demand for more extensive yet cheaper health care for everyone. On the other, there is the imperative to question what resources we can knowingly commit to the task of keeping Americans of all ages alive and healthy for as long as possible.

Nowhere is this dilemma reflected more dramatically than in the long-term care setting. Each day those of us in both institutional and community-based long-term care struggle with issues that extend far beyond what is superficially called "pulling the plug." For example, when, if ever, should life-prolonging treatment be terminated? Who should make this decision, and how should it be made? How do we help family members and caregivers from all disciplines deal with the anguish they feel in grappling with these issues? How do we properly address decisions near the end of life for people who can no longer communicate and who have left us no advance directives? Can we educate the American population—and the elderly in particular—to the need for advance directives? Can we, as a society, economically afford to continue to provide unlimited medical treatment for growing numbers of severely demented elderly? Is it ethical to develop public policies stating when care can be terminated?

Last year, a well-known woman sat at the bedside of her father as he lay dying in a hospital after suffering a stroke. "When does life start?" she asked. "When does life end? Who should be making these life-and-death decisions?" The woman was Hillary Rodham Clinton, and the grief and agony associated with those questions were no less difficult for the First Lady than they are for the rest of us. And every day, in hospitals, nursing homes, and hospices throughout this country we struggle with these issues.

As Dr. Libow noted in the Introduction to this book, the chapters in this volume are derived from presentations given at a conference on ethics and long-term care. The conference, titled "Doing the Right Thing: Grappling with the Ethical Dilemmas in Geriatric Long-term Care," focused on some of the most perplexing ethical dilemmas facing those of us who live and work in long-term care settings. Hopefully, this book sheds some light on these most difficult issues, providing new perspectives and some comfort to long-term care practitioners as we struggle together to do the right thing for our patients, their families, and ourselves.

# Index